THE FROG LETTERS

DianaRae

WingSpan Press

Unless otherwise noted, scripture quotations come from THE HOLY
BIBLE, NEW INTERNATIONAL VERSION®, NIV® Copyright ©
1973, 1978, 1984, 2011 by Biblica, Inc.™ Used by permission.

All rights reserved worldwide.

Published in the United States and the United Kingdom

by WingSpan Press, Livermore, CA

The WingSpan name, logo and colophon are the trademarks of
WingSpan Publishing.

ISBN 978-1-59594-506-8 (pbk.)

ISBN 978-1-59594-850-2 (ebk.)

First edition 2013

Printed in the United States of America

www.wingspanpress.com

Library of Congress Control Number: 2013953338

1 2 3 4 5 6 7 8 9 10

This book is dedicated to:

Those who walked before us,
those who walked with us,
and those who've yet to walk
cancer's path.

*

Andy and Donna,
for lifting her up as
she walked through the valley.

The following book is based on a true story.

Preface

On April 25, 2010, a lone figure set out on a nightly stroll through a south Arlington, Texas, neighborhood. The path, over the course of two weeks, had become familiar. One house stood out from the rest. It was a cute, pink-brick home with a well-manicured yard and a brick mailbox adorned with a small, green ceramic frog on top. Each night, the lady would watch for this house that marked the halfway point on her walk. Occasionally, the frog was moved to a new spot as if the homeowners sensed it grew bored. It was because of this, she believed they must love this frog. On this night, in the mere seconds it took for her hand to reach out for the frog, tucking it close to her, lives would forever change as she continued her walk with company.

The following day, the frog's picture was taken on top the sign for John Peter Smith's Center for Cancer Care in Fort Worth, Texas. Hours later, the frog would mail his first letter and picture home to his family. . . with no return address.

Keeping identities and location secret the duration of these writings, this is a collection of letters narrated by the frog to his family. Initially, these letters were not written with the intent of publication. Years would pass before the frog was reunited with his family. This is a true story of one family reaching out to complete strangers by sharing the most personal aspects of their lives as a cancer journey unfolds.

APRIL 26, 2010

Dear Family,

    I'm sure, by now, you've noticed I'm gone. Please don't be mad at me, but I've decided to spend time with a family who has a sister and brother with cancer. I'm sure I can bring them some joy during this time.

    Please don't try to find me. I promise I'll write as often as I can and I'll be back before you know it.

Love,

Your Frog

          ◆   ◆   ◆   ◆   ◆   ◆   ◆   ◆

APRIL 30, 2010

Dear Family,

I'll tell you about the Lady's family (where I'm staying). The Brother moved in with the Sister so she could take care of him. Two months ago, he had radical surgery because of cancer. The back bone of his leg was used to reconstruct his jaw. He looks fine to me, so don't worry; I'm not scared. This was his first week of radiation treatment so we drove to the John Peter Smith (JPS) Cancer Center every day and sometimes twice a day. He has five more weeks to go and then his treatments are finished!

The Sister doesn't feel well at all. They found out last week that she's had cancer for at least five years. Everyone is upset because of this news. She has to have some tests run before her treatments begin. Her doctor said she'll have both chemo and radiation treatments at the same time.

There's another person—the Lady. The Lady is who brought me home with her. She's the older sister (just barely, she told me to say) to the Brother and Sister and she came here to take care of them. The Lady loves them a lot.

Did you know radiation patients having the same type treatment as the Brother need fake saliva? The Lady went to fill the Brother's prescription this week. Four boxes of fake saliva cost $695. The Lady offered to spit in his mouth for a bargain price of $500, but he didn't think that was funny at all!

I'll write soon.

Yours,

Frog

♦ ♦ ♦ ♦ ♦ ♦ ♦ ♦

MAY 7, 2010

Dear Family,

The Sister is ill. For weeks now, the Lady and Brother leave her behind as they go to his treatments or appointments. She feels sad she's no longer able to be the Brother's caretaker, shadow, handholder, protector, and cheerleader. With reluctance, the Sister has relinquished these duties to the Lady and waits each day for their return as they report details of their day to her.

The Lady feels anxious. Treatment for the Sister is taking a while to begin. Nearly every day, she enters the clinic and crosses the familiar linoleum path that leads to the Sister's cancer doctor, all the while fearful of the reception she'll receive when the woman at the window recognizes her—the "pest."

She steps up to the glass window with her Bible cradled in her left arm, places her purse on the counter, and clinches her fist around a tissue with her right hand. With dread of the answer she'll get today (or won't get), she inquires if anything has been scheduled. Words are exchanged that sound foreign coming from her lips—words like *deteriorating*. Phrases that used to be a good thing are now the enemy as she leans over the counter and whispers, "losing weight." Open desperation takes her voice hostage as she reminds them, once again, five years sneaked by with no warning. She feels they were ambushed! No fair! No fair! It's as if life broke an unthinkable rule. They're an organized family—preparers. If only they'd known, they could have prepared—would, in fact, have prepared. The Lady's voice catches each time, as she fights for composure, wondering at what point in this short journey she became such a crybaby. Normally, she's strong. No news again today. Slowly, the Lady makes her way to the radiation department and we take a seat to wait for the Brother. She'll lift, as she does most every day, the soft, velvet bookmark revealing where she left off the day before and begin to read her Bible. Occasionally, she'll lift her eyes. Scanning the room, she'll make eye contact with

DianaRae

someone. They'll bond with no words. Yes, we're here—you and me. Cancer has united us for this moment. Tomorrow? Yes, we'll speak again then.

She'll daydream about years to come when this is but a distant memory, still seen clearly, yet not so painful. Perhaps they'll win the lotto. They don't need all of it—just some. They'll go back to the days when they were able to buy the large-size vanilla lattes from the Quick Stop. Together they'll raise their red paper cups in the air, pressing the plastic lids together in a salute to them—the Brother, Sister, and Lady—three siblings.

Yours,

Frog

♦ ♦ ♦ ♦ ♦ ♦ ♦ ♦

MAY 11, 2010

Dear Family,

Last week, we were driving to the cancer center and there was a drunk driver behind us. We were on Rosedale where there's stop-and-go traffic. An officer was coming toward us so the Lady spastically flapped her arm out the window and did a "thumbs back" sign pointing to the car behind us. (Yes, this is bona fide proof I'm staying with a big, fat tattletaler.) Once the officer pulled a U-turn and got behind that car, the driver became a model citizen with impeccable driving skills—almost award-winning. Never mind that earlier the Lady observed that car driving on the concrete median, repeatedly swerving into oncoming traffic. The officer tailgated the car through several stoplights before turning on her lights and pulling the car over. The Lady calls it the "intimidation factor." Whenever she's been tailgated by a law enforcement officer, her driving skills fly out the window. Where previously she was driving in complete control with one finger barely on the steering wheel, she is then forced to grip the steering wheel so tightly that her knuckles turn white as she wrestles the unruly beast of a machine to keep it under control. Her right leg uncontrollably shakes and her foot begins to thump in a nervous twitch that causes sporadic quick bursts of acceleration. This is much the same reaction her body has when she dresses inappropriately on a bitter cold day and ends up being stuck outside to brave the elements. The Lady becomes so unnerved when being tailgated by police, it's all she can do not to pull over, throw her license at the officer, and demand he send her to jail—menace on the road that she is.

The Lady injured her back because she was half impatient and half showing off as she tried to lug a recliner around the room by herself. She woke up the next day loudly saying, "Uhhhh!" each time she moved. Eventually, the Brother got totally annoyed with her, I mean, look what HE survived. What's a little back injury? She confided in me she didn't know how she managed to drive because even when she applied the brakes, it hurt her back. She's better now since she's seen a chiropractor several times. It was the first time the Lady ever had her neck popped. She wished someone was there to witness it because she convinced herself, years ago, if anyone ever attempted that procedure, her neck would snap resulting in instant death or an equally disturbing outcome—permanently injuring her and possibly even severing her spinal cord, resulting in paralysis.

Friday night, the Lady's two sons arrived to check on her to make sure she was really okay and not just saying that for their sakes. Also, they wanted to see the Brother and Sister. We went out to dinner at Abuelos. It's a gorgeous restaurant. I had enchiladas and the sopapillas were exceptional! The service was great. When I get home, we should go there for dessert.

I'll write soon!

Yours,

Frog

♦ ♦ ♦ ♦ ♦ ♦ ♦ ♦

MAY 14, 2010

Dear Family,

The Parents of the siblings are planning a trip to check on their kids. They will travel far to do this. All paraphernalia has been hidden. Paraphernalia includes a decent variety of candy bars, fresh glazed donuts, and the Lady's personal favorite—a two-inch long wafer-like hollow tube cookie with a thin vanilla frosting coated inside. They're an excellent source for a workout because the slightest provocation of lip contact causes them to crumble into hundreds of tiny flakes, making it necessary to do a series of leg squats to retrieve them off the floor. It's for this exact reason the Lady's not going to be lazy about the whole thing and simply eat them over the sink!

All of the hiding is in anticipation of "the talk." They imagine a powwow held in the living room to discuss everyone's nutritional well-being. This talk will be serious. Therefore, all the out-of-control-hyena-snorting-laughing of which they've been guilty, while lounging on comfortable chairs in the garage, will cease and be replaced with the more mature laugh reserved for public and parent display. The Lady plans to listen while slowly tapping her index finger to her lips and hopes this passes as a serious, adult look.

The refrigerator contents have already been addressed. Thanks to countless hours spent on the floor playing with their kids' Lincoln Logs over 20 years ago, the siblings retrieved the cucumbers from the crisper and have strategically constructed a solid wall of cucumbers standing at attention to block the remnants of two nights ago when the Lady, in a cooking frenzy, whipped up chili cheese dogs with frozen fast-food fries baked and seasoned with just the right amount of too much salt. Individual serving cups of fruit, applesauce, jello, and pudding now form a tower of intricate design blocking additional questionable contents. Everyone's been warned—sampling the tower goods is now off limits!

The Lady's turned into the juice police. Everyone is happy with the cheap one that, technically, has only five percent juice content. It's the other 95 percent of the content they find so darn tasty! Then there's the special juice that's the best of them all, but costs practically "an arm and a leg" for one bottle. The organic blueberry pomegranate is the REAL deal—the "Holy Grail" of all juices. The Lady walks around reminding others that the special juice is for the cancer patients. Then she makes mysterious trips to the laundry room to down shots of it, only to return seconds later, walking quickly and toting a hand towel as a diversion while wiping her wrist across her lips.

The Brother, after proofreading what I've written so far, announced this was, "Way out there! WAY out there!" He simply doesn't see how I, an uneducated frog, could be writing this. So, duly insulted, I will close for now.

Yours,

Frog

♦ ♦ ♦ ♦ ♦ ♦ ♦ ♦

MAY 19, 2010

Dear Family,

Lately, I've had a guilty conscience because of how abruptly I left. Perhaps you're wanting me home and have no way to contact me . . .

If this is ever the case, please tie the enclosed yellow ribbon around the ol', um, mailbox flag.

Miss you,

Frog

◆ ◆ ◆ ◆ ◆ ◆ ◆ ◆

MAY 22, 2010

Dear Family,

In one of the siblings' more meaningful garage-lounging conversations, they veered off discussing the merits of Chuck E.Cheese. None of them could recall exactly which decade they had last visited the place. The Lady added her two cents worth on how many times her kids' birthday parties were held at the one right here in Arlington. Her oldest nephew (son to the Sister) got a pained, faraway look on his face then quietly said he'd always wished for a birthday at Chuck E. Cheese. The Lady felt mortified and thoughtless—forgetting that although the Sister was a single parent and a good provider, Chuck E. Cheese birthday celebrations were slightly out of reach.

On May 18, 2010, the oldest nephew turned 30 years old by celebrating at Chuck E. Cheese. Let the record show, it's never too late to grab hold of a wish and make it a reality.

Yours,

Frog

♦ ♦ ♦ ♦ ♦ ♦ ♦ ♦

JUNE 1, 2010

Dear Family,

I apologize for not writing sooner; it was a really, really bad week for my adopted family. No good news to report, but I will tell you more in my next letter. Well, on second thought, there *was* a speck of good news. On Saturday, the Lady finally decided to do something with her hair. It's been put on the back burner for months now. All I can say is thank goodness!

Oh, one more thing, the Cavalry (the Mom and Dad) arrived. They love me already—but what's not to love, right? (wink wink)

Love,

Your Frog

♦ ♦ ♦ ♦ ♦ ♦ ♦ ♦

JUNE 5, 2010

Dear Family,

The Sister started chemo and radiation. The siblings' lives will never quite fit the same mold. Shattered routines lay littered—a former remnant of their previously orderly life. Radiation has nearly been conquered by the Brother. Chemo is the unknown. The Sister, wearing a portable pouch around her waist with a tube leading to a port in her chest, has chemicals released into her body every few seconds for 24 hours a day. The comfort of their security now lays within the very walls they previously couldn't have escaped from fast enough.

Two days later, with the Sister becoming sicker each day, the Lady's beside herself with worry as they maneuver the route leading to chemo. Treatment is halted. Instructions are issued to go to the hospital as the Sister's blood pressure plummets and she lies weak and nauseous. It's there she'll remain for eight days. Her body, locked up with chills and uncontrollable shaking, is layered with blankets. Feeling tremors raging through her as she struggles for warmth, the Lady does the first thing that comes to mind, she places her head on the Sister's chest and snuggles up next to her. It makes her wonder if moments such as these are what true sisterly love means. Yes. She's convinced it is.

Later, blankets are thrown off after the Lady watches the Sister's temperature climb alarmingly high. Behind the Sister's back, she'll motion to the nurse by placing a finger to her own lips as a code for silence—a secret shared between the two. *Please don't tell her! It'll frighten her!*

There will always be those moments that impact our lives—forever changing them or their course—memories that refuse to weaken with time. Lies will be revealed. Beloved pets will be put down. A promise will be kept when you were expecting it to be broken. Strong fathers will hang their heads and weep in defeat while pleading to someone, anyone, yet no one really, *"Someone has to SAVE her!"* Mothers will stand in the background, wringing their hands, numb with pain over sick children. A sister will quietly recall a particular cemetery she always admired while passing. Words spoken out loud that can't be taken back—the ones you never want to hear, because that's the rule. Did you know this? As long as it's never said out loud, it isn't so.

Two-second eye contact will be shared with a complete stranger you somehow recognize. A page will be torn and carelessly thrown away, forever gone, never to be put back in place again.

Yours,

Frog

♦ ♦ ♦ ♦ ♦ ♦ ♦ ♦

JUNE 8, 2010

Dear Family,

One day, the Lady stood in the radiation waiting area as the Brother and Sister sat waiting for treatment. She told how she was getting sick herself. Three nights in a row she had stepped out of the shower to face the mirror only to discover a very large, round, red circle on her stomach. After investigating it closely (without touching it) she grimly determined it must be a ringworm. I mean, what else could it be all "ringy-looking"? Why didn't she ever notice it during the day? Was this contagious? She would need to do a little Internet research in private.

Well, she fretted for days about how she would break it to her siblings since they use the same shower. Why couldn't she just have a canker sore? Anything with the word *worm* attached to it just sounded so... *wormy*. (She stared hard at the ring for several moments to try to catch any signs of movement or variation in formation.) Was it angry-looking today versus yesterday? She couldn't tell. Would the siblings be understanding? Would she be if the tables were turned? In a split second she knew the answer was NO! Convinced if one of the siblings disclosed that a case of ringworm was running rampant throughout the household, she would be taking all future showers while wearing four-inch heels! Silently, she congratulated herself on being so perceptive in having already solved any possible future contamination issues involving *that*. She would be totally prepared now. Totally!

By far, the biggest area of concern would be the medical expense involved in getting rid of it. The Lady only has hospitalization insurance so she wonders exactly how long she'll need to turn a "blind eye" until it's officially big enough to require hospitalization so it's covered, yet, not ridiculously large where it would start screwing around with body parts that are mandatory for her survival.

Obviously, the Internet research is going to be more extensive than she had originally thought.

By this time, the Brother and Sister are absorbed in the story; it appears they are leaning further back in their chairs as a contamination precaution the Lady both recognizes and appreciates. Hysterical laughter breaks out as the Lady confides in them. She finally realized the large, round ring was the result of changing her shower routine after she injured her back. It was easier to shove the shaving cream can hard against her stomach for fast dispensing, thus creating the ring!

Yours,

Frog

♦ ♦ ♦ ♦ ♦ ♦ ♦ ♦

JUNE 12, 2010

Dear Family,

Good news this time! Yesterday, the Brother finished seven straight weeks of radiation. We were all there to be with him, but I turned into a special guest. No one, and I mean no one, well . . . *hardly* anyone, is allowed back in radiation. That door has always been so mysterious to me. The closest I've gotten was when the Sister was in the hospital and after a few days, when she was stable enough to move, they transported her from the hospital to the cancer center to continue her treatment. The Lady and I got to ride with her and go in through the back door. Yesterday, the Lady whispered around to some people that I was special to the family and they got authorization to clear me through the mysterious door. Can you believe that? I think it was because of Tera. She's the woman we report to each day at the front desk of the radiation department.

As we entered the first room, I was put on the table where the Brother and Sister had once lain before starting radiation treatments. Here's where the exact spots, pinpoint precision targets for radiation, were tattooed on the siblings in ink. After that, we went through this very heavy vault-like door. From this point on it's totally serious business. Hello! We're talkin' radiation! This door is shut behind the patients as soon as they clear it.

You wind your way down this hallway where the walls are lead-lined as a protection from the inner treatment room where one patient at a time is allowed. This is where the Brother received his treatments. I checked to see if the Lady was getting emotional. Music played softly in this room at that moment. It reminded me of the one time we entered through the back door with the Sister. While the Sister was having her treatment, the Lady heard music swell to this wonderfully loud crescendo causing her to rise from her chair and press her palm to her chest. It was angel music and she was getting to share this moment with her sister—a moment knowing that whatever the

Sister was experiencing on the other side of those lead-lined walls—hopefully, it was going to make her well.

The Brother brought a souvenir home. It was his face mask that was molded to his face before he started treatment. It looks friendly but he says it's not because it's strapped to the table so he can't move. The Lady investigates it more closely and recalls one day, several weeks into treatment, they were driving home when the Brother announced his face mask used to fit tight and snug against his face; however, he was noticing there was more room in it now. "Radiation must be shrinking my head!" the Brother said. The Lady did a mental visual on how, perhaps eventually, his head would be the size of a tomato!

Yours,

Frog

♦   ♦   ♦   ♦   ♦   ♦   ♦   ♦

JUNE 14, 2010

Dear Family,

Today is Monday, June 14, 2010. The household has moved from Level Orange to Level Red. The Sister is to start chemo again today. Anxiety fills the air as the portable chemo pouch is retrieved and placed on the table so it's not forgotten.

People ask what the difference is between *chemo* and *radiation*. The short of it is, radiation targets a specific area released by a laser beam. Chemo knows no boundaries. It travels throughout the body killing cancer cells, so, it's a friend. However, unfortunately, it kills a person's good cells too. Therefore, chemo is also the enemy. Blood counts of patients are monitored closely because of this. I learned that cancer's not rare. Right now, over 11 ½ million people in the United States have cancer. I'm sending you a picture taken today with the radiation doctor, Dr. Hernandez, who's very nice! The Lady goofed and accidentally had the Sister in the picture so we're going to muddy that up a bit so her identity stays secret a while longer.

The Lady and I left very early this morning to travel to where she used to live. She discovered she had a cavity and actually felt happy she would get to see Dr. Glover and her "dentist family" again. You could tell she likes these people a whole lot and they like her as well.

The Lady drove out of town forgetting to ask where she could obtain one of those dentist chairs for her own personal use. She discovered today, due to the unique design, it gives off some sort of fantastic optical illusion that her stomach is flat! Yes, she needs one and has already determined it to be a worthwhile purchase. If she ever has company, she could lounge around portraying ignorance that anything concave looking may be happening at her mid-section!

(Later in the day.) Chemo has been stopped for the Sister until her last week of radiation. Everyone's very relieved and we celebrated by eating just way too much! The siblings' Parents will leave in the morning for their long journey home. I'll miss them—all of us will. I miss you too!

Yours,

Frog

♦　♦　♦　♦　♦　♦　♦　♦

JUNE 16, 2010

Dear Family,

This morning, the Lady was on the computer when the Sister came in from getting dressed to lay down on the bed behind her. Today is not a good day for the Sister. She's sad. She's feeling discouraged. She'll begin to talk earnestly to the Lady—spilling feelings from her heart. The Lady swivels her chair around giving the Sister her undivided attention. She takes the Sister's hand in her own and presses a kiss to it, then continues to hold it. The Sister confides she was expecting to feel better by now, but each day it becomes a little more difficult and she feels a little worse. She knows she's lost weight she couldn't really afford to lose. When she dressed this morning in front of the mirror, she saw bones protruding. Also, she was hoping her tumor would have shrunk; instead it's growing. She's so tired!

The Lady gently reminds her that her radiation just started. It's too soon! Besides, the chemo doctor told the Sister, "(Sister's name), you're going to have to fight!" Remember? They knew this wasn't going to be easy.

Is it the radiation? Is it the morphine? Which one has robbed her appetite? The Sister thinks she'll try to eliminate some of the morphine. The Lady slowly closes her eyes and keeps them closed, breathing deeply. They've been down this familiar route. It's no good—absolutely no good.

Their only hope is in Him. Hot tears trail down the Lady's face, drop, then continue their journey down the Sister's arm while the Sister's tears pour down from the sides of her eyes to become lost in her hair—that same precious hair she so fears losing with chemo. Oh, sweet Jesus!

I'm sorry, my family, but I can not continue this story. I grasp to recall the words spoken between them. Fervent prayers, feelings, and words I know I could never recapture exactly nor do justice.

You see, I was but a casual observer in that room this morning, an intruder for the moment.

Yours,

Frog

♦ ♦ ♦ ♦ ♦ ♦ ♦ ♦

JUNE 21, 2010

Dear Family,

There's a camaraderie among the people at the cancer center. No bias here. Everyone is in it together regardless of their role as the patient or caregiver. Radiation appointments are usually daily at the same time. On some days, the machine or patient will have problems and the wait may take hours. There's ample time to get to know those around you. If they're running ahead of schedule, an empty waiting room will greet you. You'll feel happy, yet disappointed at the same time.

Chemo is in one area, while radiation is in another. Rarely will you get to know anyone in chemo if you're a radiation patient. The ones who simultaneously have both, although unspoken, are held in high regard. They are the warriors. It's hard enough having one treatment let alone both. They shed some light on the unknown. Stories will be swapped, symptoms hashed out, treatments compared, and diagnoses feared. The Sister becomes ill listening to such talk. However, there's also comfort that the people among you are certifiable proof you're definitely not alone in this.

Several men share the same type cancer as the Brother but none to his extent in this group. He hobbles into the center with his cane while sporting a new jaw–compliments of the back bone of his leg. Who came up with that concept? Who was that very first person who said, *"Why yes! I do believe I'm crafty enough to tackle this! I'll just take the old, rotten bone out, borrow some good bone from over there, whittle it a little here and a little there, stick the new one in and there you have it!"* The Brother's facial structure remains hardly changed. Yes, it's unbelievable. Surgeons deserve standing ovations for such bravado.

The Brother's treatments, normally in the afternoon, ended with a morning appointment. We all filtered in, taking seats together in a row, except for the Dad who ventured around the corner to sit a while in the doctors' waiting room. Strangers were among us. Our friends are not here to witness this momentous occasion.

A short time later, a woman arrives with a mentally-challenged young man in tow. We've never seen them before. They take seats directly in front of us. She tells us she's raised her nephew since he was a toddler so they always make this trip together. Her appointment is early today, as well, and normally she knows others here who will watch him while she has treatment. She asks if we would mind watching him. The Lady immediately replies, "No worries!" The Lady has already taken a liking to her nephew. He is shy and sweet. The woman points out a small gift sack he carries that holds a variety of pictures he likes to look at. There's also a container of jumbo Legos.

Eventually, the Dad joins the group, taking a seat among the family. The woman's name is called. Right on cue, the Lady leaves her seat and crosses over to sit with the woman's nephew. The Lady reaches for the gift bag, drawing it to her, she peers into the bag and starts to finger the contents. Saying in an overly excited voice, "Why! What've you got in this bag?" Immediately, the Dad snaps at her in his stern voice used to reprimand, "It's none of your *business* what he has in his bag!" Everyone breaks out laughing, realizing he missed "the drill" by sitting in the other room and was clueless of the plan. Knowing the Lady so well, the Brother says the Dad probably thought she was searching for candy!

Yours,

Frog

♦ ♦ ♦ ♦ ♦ ♦ ♦ ♦

JUNE 24, 2010

Dear Family,

The Lady and I were on a quest the other day. The printer was out of ink. My letter to you was like a festering wound, sitting unprinted in the documents file on the computer. It was equally important that we print out a head shot to muddy up that picture of the Sister and Dr. Hernandez. We drove to four major retailers, but no one carried the ink cartridge we needed. The Lady was calm about it, but I was getting very frustrated. It took me forever to type that letter! However, the Lady is pretty innovative. We drove to a fast food restaurant off Sublett Road. There was a lull in the place, with a few patrons. It was between lunch and dinner time. The Lady explained to the girl at the counter that she needed a small head shot of Jack—preferably in color and on paper (expecting there to be a ready stack of them under the counter in the event anyone, such as us, were to walk in and request one). The girl searched anything in the area that could meet our requirements. Nope! Nothing. Now, granted, they *do* have a gift card in color that, if push comes to shove, might work. However, it would be quite difficult to cut that head off hard plastic. Certainly, it would lack the effect we were striving to achieve.

I took over, asking the employees to please help find any sort of head shot. *Can someone check the paper drink cups? What's on the outside? Nothing?* The kid making hamburgers snapped to attention to scan his work area–clearly a teamplayer in this fine establishment. After double-checking under the counter, he produced a perfectly packaged car antenna topper. Well, it's not quite what we had in mind, but the Lady stuffed it in her purse anyway. We left feeling really good about the employee work ethic there.

"What are you gonna do with it?" I asked a few days later, as the Lady tossed the antenna topper on the dresser.

"Why?"

"We should give it to my family. They'll remember my letter and know it's from me."

"Are you nuts? Let me get this straight. You want us to creep all the way over there in the dark, place this on their car antenna, snap a picture, then scurry off like some sort of criminal? Get back home, realize all the pictures didn't turn out due to a combination of I'm too short and my hand was shaking uncontrollably. Stew over it all night because I want the *right* picture, drive back over in the morning in an attempt to get another picture when all bravery flees me? Preposterous! What if we get caught?"

"Then I'll tell them I love and miss them, I'm fine, and I'll be home soon."

Yours,

Frog

♦ ♦ ♦ ♦ ♦ ♦ ♦ ♦

JUNE 28, 2010

Dear Family,

The portable chemo pouch is in the Lady's car. This is it. Today is *the* day. There will be no turning back or last-minute changes by the doctor this time. The atmosphere has changed considerably compared to the first attempt at chemo that ended in that eight-day hospital stay. Remember that? The Sister's attitude is one of, "Bring it on! Bring! It! On!" Oh yeah, she's ready alright. The Lady shakes her fist in the air in a sign of declared war and destined victory over this stupid cancer. We can do this! Secret fears assail her, though, as the Sister stopped all morphine well over a week ago in an attempt to get her appetite back. Decisions! Decisions! How does someone endure the pain cancer inflicts when large tumors and radiation treatments are a constant part of your daily life? I don't know. The Sister will lay curled up in one of three spots in the house at any given moment during the day. The Lady will seek her out, check on her, push food, smile over empty plates, bowls and wrappers, and feel her forehead as she sleeps. The Mom says their family is being smiled on. I'm a witness. I tell you this is so.

Last Monday, the Brother had a second skin graph on his leg. Some days are busier than others. This is one of those days. The Lady dropped the Brother off at the hospital at 11:30 a.m., drove the Sister to radiation, waited as she had treatment, drove her back home, then turned around and hightailed it back to the hospital for the Brother. The three of us finally walked back through the door Tuesday at one in the morning. There were three angels working the surgery floor that night at John Peter Smith Hospital, Ft. Worth - Mary, Rick, and Cindy. While hospital administrators were tucked in beds and unaware, the nursing staff was making lives a little easier for others. With no cameras rolling, acts of kindness were going undocumented in personnel files. Compassion for others, with no ulterior motive or secret agenda, failed to be observed by superiors. We left the hospital tired but smiled upon.

For two months now, a stash of money laid untouched for the siblings—courtesy of their Aunt Bev in Tucson. Instructions were to use it for gas or whatever the Lady felt the family needed. It took no time for the Lady to realize the household needed a new range. The outer pane of their range was missing, creating much difficulty when trying to bake.

Because she hates shopping, the Lady waits for the Parents to visit. They pre-screen floor models at Sears and narrow it down to two. The following week, the Lady goes to the store and only looks at those two models. She opens the oven door on one brand, but it's heavy and catches midway through. Taking the GE oven handle in her grasp, it opens effortlessly and seems to beckon to her, *I'm friendly. Buy me.* With the decision made, the salesclerk begins to ring up the purchase—cost, tax, delivery charge, removal of the old unit, and a new adapter. "That's so strange when this happens," Harold, the salesman, says when the total appears. The Lady takes a look and can't believe it either so she shares her story with him. The grand total, to the exact penny, was the amount Aunt Bev had sent them.

On Thursday, the Sister and Lady walk into the hospital early that morning for the Sister's liver biopsy. They were already forewarned in April and May that her liver had some spots. They are ready to move her to the procedure room when the doctor asks, at the last minute, if she's seen the CT scan of her liver taken during her hospital stay. No, she hasn't. Would she like to? "Sure," the Sister replies. The doctor instructs the nurse to unhook her IV. The Sister climbs out of bed and we walk to a computer where six of us gather around as an image appears on the screen. The image shows the truth to all who look upon it in the room. The liver is in trouble. It's riddled with spots all over—large spots, small spots, dark spots, and light spots, too many to even count. The Lady and Sister don't dare look at each other for fear of what emotions will be read upon their faces. The Sister feels like crawling back in the bed and crying when she sees this. The Lady has to restrain herself, as well, from throwing herself into the nearest bed to roll around in her misery. Might as well rip her heart out now . . .

The doctor says, "You need to get back on chemo right away." Curious, the Lady asks which spot he plans to biopsy. He says it's not going to matter—whatever is in one will be in all the others. The Sister is hooked back up to the IV. The Lady walks beside the bed as the Sister is wheeled down the hallway to the procedure room, all the while issuing last-minute instructions to the Sister.

"Remember! Angels are around you! Oh, and ask God for peace!" the Lady says.

Eventually, the nurse seeks out the Lady in the waiting room. As they retrace their steps to the Sister, he apologizes for the delay. They had to move her from the ultrasound room to the CT scan room to get a better view of the liver. It seems they were hardly able to find anything to biopsy! The liver spots were hardly there. You know it! Smiled upon.

Here's what I've learned, when life picks you up and slams you down into quicksand (and we all know at some point in our lives this is going to happen), you can struggle and resist and sink under the weight of it all, or you can relax, let it go, look up, and be smiled upon.

Yours,

Frog

♦　♦　♦　♦　♦　♦　♦　♦

JULY 1, 2010

Dear Family,

The Lady let the Sister down and is disappointed in herself. She attempted to enter the chemo area for moral support and lasted just minutes before she excused herself and fled the room. There are 18 chairs filled with patients connected to pouches—pouches that are killing, pouches that are healing. She can't deal with it. She just . . . can't. Not yet. We sat in the waiting area. Periodically, the Lady rises from her chair, peeps through the small window in the door to check on the Sister, then returns to her seat. Someone wheels in a cart of wigs—free for the taking. The Sister already has a wig at home, hidden in her closet out of view, in case her own hair falls victim to the chemo. Not everyone loses their hair. At one point, the Lady considered shaving off her own hair as a bonding gesture if this happens to the Sister, but that lasted maybe a split second before she started making excuses for herself to hide her vanity.

Driving away from the cancer center on Monday made the Lady anxious. She was stressed about the chemo pump being connected to the Sister again. We had barely exited the parking lot when we heard it dispensing chemicals into the Sister every 30 seconds. The Lady turned the radio up in an attempt to drown the pump noise that, everyone agrees, sounds robotic. Then, subconsciously, she started associating the sound as some sort of time bomb which caused everything to majorly grate on her nerves. The seat belt strap became unbearable and way too restraining so she hooked a thumb under it and stretched it to the steering wheel, wrapping her hand around both, and continued driving. By the time we were on I-35, her saliva glands kicked in full force which meant there was half a chance or better she was going to be sick to her stomach. The Sister picked up on this and asked the Lady if she was okay.

The Lady answered quickly, "Yes! Fine!" She doesn't want to talk about it for fear it will promote the nausea. Emotionally shot, she

DianaRae

turned the radio volume up. (*La-la-la I can't hear you. Don't make me think right now, just institutionalize me! Whatever was I thinking? I lied! I can't do this. I'm WEAK . . . not strong.*) Devil thoughts run helter-skelter when fear invades.

Radiation continues every day for the Sister, but they have shaved four days off her treatment plan, which is a good sign. On Wednesday, we returned to chemo to have a second pouch connected that will carry her until Friday when she'll be disconnected. For how long? We don't know yet. However, pouch number one still has about three hours of chemicals left. They could open the valve and drain it through, but they don't want to do this. We're told to come back in about three hours. Getting as far as the stoplight down the road, the pump makes a noise none of us has heard before. The Lady snaps the radio off with lightening speed. Ears strain for a repeat sound. Hearts race. The Sister unzips the fanny pack and takes the pump/time bomb out to have a look. The Lady has already determined it to be unfriendly because she prefers anything computerized have two options: On or Off. The Sister presses the Off button, the On button, and it starts filtering information on the screen. Traffic forces the Lady to continue making a left turn onto Rosedale. Traffic is thick. The Sister asks if she should press Yes or No for a question on the screen that sounds suspiciously to the Lady like a scientist should be answering it, certainly not her!

We bottom out in the car while making a fast turn around and head back to the cancer center. The sisters are becoming hysterical by discussing perhaps the wrong button *was* pushed and now it's dispensing chemicals at a ridiculously rapid rate. For the love of . . . someone call an ambulance! Reaching the parking lot entrance, all the while counting seconds between each pump dispensing, they determine the pump is working perfectly. Afterward, they laugh for a long time about the shear madness they just shared.

So far, so good with the Sister and her chemo this week. All the dooo-dooo dooo-dooo (theme from *Jaws* music) preconceived notions of a repeat of last time have not yet materialized. So, what's to eat around here? Let's celebrate!

Love,

Frog

JULY 7, 2010

Dear Family,

The Brother hasn't eaten this year. He's still fed through a feeding tube in his stomach. He desperately wants food and has now lost over 100 pounds. Cases of Carnation Breakfast and Boost were organized on the pantry shelf. Flavors include chocolate, vanilla, and strawberry—none enticing. Flavors are irrelevant because anything that goes into the tube has zero taste. Gatorade is chosen by the Lady according to what color it is, whether it strikes her as a pleasant shade at that moment. Gone are the days when she bothered pulling out her reading glasses to actually see what flavor she was buying. The real world of food doesn't exist much for the Brother.

Full of sympathy, their oldest sister Donna (who lives in New Jersey and visited a couple months back) proudly presented him with a nice plate of hot scrambled eggs, soft and just the right texture, a love gesture gone sour after he put the first bite in his mouth and yelled in pain. Panic ensued. *Quick! Spit it out! Spit it out!* As if those are magic words that will somehow undo the damage. Weeks later, the Lady accompanied him for an exam and told the doctor of the incident. The Lady ended up being slightly reprimanded for trying to make his jaw work when it's still too early. This almost embarrassed me to death!

It would be realistic to say the Brother keeps a mental list of grievances against the Lady when it comes to his food experiences. Grievance #1: The Brother explicitly instructed the Lady, "Under no circumstance should you release the firm grip you have holding the feeding tube and large syringe together, like this, in one hand. SEE? Are you paying attention? Quit twirling your hair! Now then, pour the stuff in with your other hand, like this." Maybe three days into the Lady's "training" she decided one morning that the first step wasn't really necessary. There's a much nicer feel to holding the top of the syringe pinched between her thumb and forefinger, pinkie out, as if she were sipping tea from fine china, THEN pour. Oh it worked alright, maybe seconds, before the syringe separated from the line and a sticky mess showered over everything, including the Brother.

Grievance #2: The Lady was in the habit of expressing if something were particularly tasty to her by saying, "Mmmm," while chewing. Victory! She has now been broken of that habit. Cured— all by a couple hateful looks pointed in her direction. She's gone the extra mile, though, by occasionally saying loud enough for him to hear, "This tastes like crap!" when it doesn't. Or, with her voice laced in disgust, "I'm *certainly* not enjoying *this*!" as she devours her Subway (ham and American, loaded) in record time.

However, she makes it up to him. Prior to her arrival, he was limited to chocolate, strawberry, and vanilla shakes. One day, the Lady stumbled upon Bruster's. Gone is the milkshake humdrum existence! They create special flavors just for the Brother. We're giving you our frequent buyer card we earned for a free shake. The Brother's favorite flavor is coffee swirl. So, try one of those, okay?

Yours,

Frog

◆ ◆ ◆ ◆ ◆ ◆ ◆ ◆

JULY 10, 2010

Dear Family,

According to Donna, it's *dimes* from heaven—not pennies. The story she's told for years now is referred to as her "dime story." She travels the world and dimes will appear in her path. You know how sometimes you just know something? When something goes so way beyond the most obvious? Donna will tell you with absolute conviction that these dimes are from heaven. Absorbed in the telling of various places dimes have shown up, there's no doubt to her they are heaven-sent—a sign she is not walking alone. The Lady, for that matter, doesn't doubt either as goosebumps appear on her arms while she listens. Donna will pick up a dime, give it a kiss, place it in her pocket, and say, "Thank you, Jesus!" Shiny dimes, real eye-catchers! She marvels at His timing in high-traffic areas where they're strategically placed, not too soon and not too late, just in time for Donna only.

Dimes, huh? Yes! Why not? I believe!

This story comes to mind now because the Lady and I have been stumbling upon dimes in our path. One time, in the cancer center parking lot, right there in clear view of foot traffic, was a dime. It should have been picked up by someone, but it was shining like a beacon to us. We stepped over it, gave it a moment's thought (dime story?), then forgot it even existed until another day, there was another brilliantly shiny dime right there on the sidewalk entering the Quick Stop. This dime is given even more thought than the last dime (Dime story? Dime story!), but is still walked over and left behind.

Last Sunday, the Lady sat in a comfortable garage chair staring at nothing, but thinking a lot about something weighing on her mind. An old aquaintance had entered her life again. What to do? What to do? Should she gather her nerve and agree to meet him? There was dead silence in the garage, no movement. That's why we both jumped when a noise sounded next to us. The Lady's first thought was someone had just thrown something in the garage! Was she the intended target? (Translated: Should she run in the house because she's no fighter?) Her eyes scanned the area by her chair since that's where the noise had originated. Looking down, to the right of the chair, laid a lone dime. She picked it up, dropped it from mid-air, and the same earlier sound filled the air, a dropped dime—from nowhere. Her eyes scanned the ceiling directly above us. Hmmm, from heaven then, for her. Picking the dime up, she raced into the house, slamming the door in haste, and spilled the story to the Sister. What does it mean? Meet him? Yes? No? Yes? No? Eeenie, meanie, miney, moe? The Sister tells her to pray about it.

(Days later . . .) There'll be no meeting. The Lady knows this in her heart to be true. Exhaling loudly and moving a little slower now, she picks up the garage dime from her dresser and puts it away for safekeeping, a reminder she listened.

WHAT? Is she NUTS? What was she thinking? He was cute! She should definitely meet him! Just see him once more in her lifetime for curiosity's sake. Yes, that's what she'll do.

Her heart wages war with her head. Nah. The heart speaks louder and wins. She will stand firm and scratch all possible future fictional scenarios she had conjured up in her mind. No future there. No settling!

Yours,

Frog

P. S. Thanks for keeping the antenna topper on your car. We drove by and checked!

♦ ♦ ♦ ♦ ♦ ♦ ♦ ♦

Dear Family,

I have good news, bad news, then some more bad news.

The Sister finished all her radiation last week so we took some boxes of cookies for the staff on her final day. With her making it through four full days of chemo, yes, she's classified as "warrior" status now!

On Friday, the Dad had a tumor removed and they were told that afternoon it was cancerous. That makes three immediate family members in four months to become victims. At first, the Sister and Lady started crying. The Sister recalls how the Dad pulled her aside when he was here to say, "Teensy, if I could take this from you in your place, I would." Wasn't that precious of him? This caused the sisters to cry even harder. They love their Dad so much and won't find out until next week what his treatment, if any, will be. They began to give thanks by talking back and forth about how lucky their family has been and how they just keep being provided for. The Lady left the room for a moment, to transfer clothes from the washer into the dryer, when the Sister and I heard her yell. She walked back (proof pinched between her fingers) saying a lone, shiny dime was in the washer, not another single coin, just the dime. The Sister says it's confirmation they're being heard.

The Lady says it's clear the family is either having their faith strengthened or they're under attack. If it's the latter, obviously *they* don't know who they're messin' with!

Now, I don't want you to get upset with the next bit of news. I want you to know that I'm fine, honestly, I am! However, for the past year or so, my right eye has been bothering me. I never got a chance to tell you this and I'm sorry. This past weekend I asked the Lady if she'd take a look at it. She assured me this was not the end of the world, but there's about a 50/50 chance I'm going to lose my right eye. She thinks it's some condition called erosion, whatever that is, and probably weather-related. She said to tell you she'll do everything in her power to prevent this from happening. Anyway, I felt you should know.

That's it for here.

Yours,

Frog

♦ ♦ ♦ ♦ ♦ ♦ ♦ ♦

Dear Family,

A pretty quiet weekend here. The Lady and I did some running around on Saturday to get supplies for the fellow residents here. Then, we zipped to the Parks Mall where I saw her wrestle with her conscience over a particularly fabulous Coach purse she wants. It got crazy watching her put it on her shoulder, look in the mirror, set it down, only to repeat the process. Her face clearly revealing that, yes, this glitzy gold/silver purse just screams her name! What *is* it about that purse? The silver disco ball thing hanging off it that's just so totally oddball that now she loves it to death? YES!! Ughhh! I just can't justify the purchase, she says. Exhaling loudly, she wonders why she has to be such a *justifiable* person! Right now, it feels like a genetic defect.

We lunched at Chick-fil-A where the "EAT MOR CHIKIN" cow was visiting. I wanted to go meet her but the Lady (after looking left then right) said, "My word! We couldn't *possibly!*" The place was a packed zoo with everyone three feet tall and under vying for her attention. I think the Lady guiltily remembered my eye condition, after I mentioned it might be the only time I'll ever *see* the cow, and decided to brave the crowd for me. I tried to make small talk but the cow doesn't speak! She only shakes her head yes or no. Yeah! No lie.

The Lady's ex-father-in-law of 25 years passed away on Friday. That made her sad. Once upon a time, she was his only caregiver too. Taking care of family—a fast-forwarded film of her life would show her doing exactly this, for always, child, spouse, parent, grandparent, and now siblings. Maybe this is, or has been all along, her purpose, her true calling, her reason for being. She's good at this. Someday when this is all over (and someday it WILL be all over), perhaps she'll ask the world, "Who needs me now?"

Yours,

Frog

◆ ◆ ◆ ◆ ◆ ◆ ◆ ◆

JULY 22, 2010

Dear Family,

The Sister cries at the drop of a hat lately. Yesterday, she asked the Lady what was wrong with her. Had she noticed how much she's crying lately? The Lady has noticed it's more frequent and tells her it's probably just menopause. Granted, it's probably not, but she's discovered you can blame practically anything at all on menopause. Spilled juice spots left on the floor of the laundry room to dry? Menopause! Neglected toe nails? Menopause! Strong desire to purchase Coach purse with disco ball ornament hanging off it? Again, menopause! The great thing about the whole menopause thing is people usually accept this (*Hmmm . . . menopause you say? Well, of COURSE it is!*) as a plausible excuse reciprocated with a good degree of sympathy.

One morning, the Sister poured her coffee, set the cup on the counter, and told the Lady in a dejected voice, "I'm so sorry you have to do so much around here." Then she broke into tears. The Lady doesn't feel like she does all that much. Heavens! She's forever indebted to the Sister for letting her be with her during all this.

Letters will arrive for the Sister from her pen pal who wonders why she doesn't write as often. This person doesn't know she's ill. Hundreds upon hundreds of people know she's ill, but one person in the Sister's life, who means a lot to her and her to him, doesn't know this. She doesn't want him to worry, she says. So she cries for fear he might be mad at her. Another day, she'll tell the Lady if anything were to happen, please write and let him know. Overcome with tears, she speaks words you never want to say out loud. Remember those? The Lady will lay in bed at night composing imaginary letters to this pen pal in her head, crying and thinking about how the Sister is the most selfless person she's ever known, always concerned about others.

Gone are the days when the Lady placed her hand on the Sister's back and said, "there there," in a soothing tone to comfort her. Nowadays, the Lady immediately advances to the tissue box, grabbing a couple in her hand and passing one to the Sister, then proceeds to join in the crying. They'll tell each other things they probably never would have under normal circumstances—secrets they planned to take to their graves, but think better of it now. It's very bonding, therapeutic, and sisterly. However, it's also this huge gut-wretching ball of emotions running unorganized all over the place that can make you sick to your stomach or bring comfort all in a matter of minutes.

So with dread of hearing, and tissues clutched in fists when noses aren't being wiped, the Sister gives the Lady explicit instructions if something *were* to happen. This is odd timing now since she seems so much stronger. Where did this foreboding come from? She recalls when their offices at work moved location last year and how she felt something inside that told her she wouldn't be there for long. Just this "feeling." Or maybe it's because the doctor told her even though her liver biopsy came out well, that doesn't necessarily mean cancer hasn't metastasized. I know, tests can tease you into false security. The Lady listens to these instructions and takes her words seriously— etching them not only into her brain but into her heart, as well, for safekeeping so they never become lost.

The next day, unbeknown to the Sister, we search the service road along 287 to find the cemetery she had mentioned. Pulling into the drive, we get out of the car and walk to the gate to peer inside. As I recall what a gentle spirit the Sister is, my one good eye becomes watery with the view; the Lady's eyes become afflicted, too. It's lovely, peaceful, and shady here. I hear the Lady take a really deep breath, exhale, and realize we both see exactly!

Love,

Your Frog

P.S. We have to make a fast trip, soon, to where the Parents live. The Lady wants to see what's going on with the Dad before treatments start here again. I promise to write and I'll be back before you know it!

♦ ♦ ♦ ♦ ♦ ♦ ♦ ♦

JULY 23, 2010

Dear Family,

The Lady and I drove forever yesterday . . .

We stopped at a casino in Shreveport, Louisiana. She brought two rolls of quarters with us and said when they were gone, so were we. We finally found the quarter slots, but couldn't find anywhere on the machines to insert the quarters and had to ask for assistance. A true gambler the Lady is not. Neither one of us had any idea that quarter slot machines no longer take quarters—only bills. Don't you find this odd? The Lady stuck a $10 in the machine and was down to her last $1.25 when it paid out very, very nicely. Nice enough that we cashed out and left with the Lady's purse clutched to her chest for financial protection because armed escort service was not available. Okay, well maybe not *that* huge of an amount but enough to make us smile. We're forwarding you half the winnings less our initial investment.

Don't worry about me. I'm totally safe and enjoying the trip so far. We stopped for the night in Leeds, Alabama.

Yours,

Frog

◆　◆　◆　◆　◆　◆　◆　◆

JULY 26, 2010

Dear Family,

We spent the weekend in Buford, Georgia, with the Lady's friend, Renee'. They've known each other since seventh grade. The Lady was thankful to get a chance to visit. She was tired, though, so her friend scratched plans and understood that just a quiet weekend is all that she wanted this time. Naps in the afternoon are relished and the Lady has to force herself to wake up. Well, except for the one time she raised her head and inquired of me, "Is that bacon I smell?" then sprang from the bed with the energy of a teenager.

One night, we stayed up until one in the morning on the back porch (her favorite porch in the world) as the two of them talked about life and cried while sharing sister stories. Watching them catch up on lost time, I realized how precious few are the minutes, an undeserved gift taken for granted. That's life. *Here, take these minutes. They're for you and JUST for you! They're yours. Now, be careful with them because you only get "some." Never, ever, EVER forget that when they're gone—they are truly, truly gone.*

You get it?

Love,

Frog

◆ ◆ ◆ ◆ ◆ ◆ ◆ ◆

Dear Family,

This is a pretty state (North Carolina). You'd love it here with all the trees! Even the weeds look all lush, green, and perfect.

We stayed at the Parents' house. I already met them when the Sister was in the hospital. Remember? Anyway, they loved having me here and were glad the Lady didn't have to travel all that way alone even though she's a road warrior. She sings at the top of her lungs to almost every song on the radio. In Mississippi, we were speeding along while singing a song she taught me. *Whom shall I fear? Whom shall I fear?* We were singing/yelling when the Lady noticed we were being tailgated by two state troopers and she sure feared them!

The Lady spent some time filling the Parents in on the siblings. Each and every time she mentions the Sister, the Dad's eyes fill with tears. He finds it difficult to speak. Everyone has turned 10 times more sentimental due to the circumstances. The Lady knows if he were well, he'd be with Teensy. His heart is with her now, just as the Lady's is, and the Mom's. The Sister has that effect even on me!

There's nothing the Dad wouldn't do for any of his kids. For instance, when the Lady first arrived, he said he believed he needed to get her that Coach purse. Right away the Lady told him, no, it wasn't necessary, but she was raised to obey (biblical principles and all) her parents. So say, if *ordered* to, she may very well be *forced* to go to Coach to buy that purse! However, the Mom says to him, "Better ask how much the purse is first." Totally, like, RUINING the whole thing! (Just kidding, honest, I am!)

We're heading back to Texas soon.

Love,

Your Frog

♦ ♦ ♦ ♦ ♦ ♦ ♦ ♦

AUGUST 4, 2010

Dear Family,

After maneuvering through Atlanta's traffic, we started making some great time getting home until we crossed into Alabama. In Alabama, the speed limit changed to 55 mph, forcing everyone to coast down to 65. This speed limit makes no sense since it's all a rural, low-traffic area and there's nothing to hit but a bunch of trees. The Lady said she figures it's to discourage people from considering moving there. Is the Governor even aware of the unwelcoming feeling this speed limit generates? It remains 55 for so ridiculously long, you get annoyed about the wrongness of it. Oh, eventually it posts 70 mph, but just when you're about to forgive and forget, and actually start feeling friendly toward Alabama (because you're back to making excellent time again and they have a good radio station), it drops back to 55! Ugh!!!!

By the time we drove across Alabama, Mississippi, and nearly all of Louisiana, the Lady's right leg was cramping up and she wasn't at all sure she'd be able to walk if we got out of the car.

We pulled off somewhere in east Texas at a Denny's. The Lady did a series of leg lunges (unintentionally) then gulped a massive amount of coffee. We got back on the road and coasted into Arlington where we slept like babies.

Inspired by a thoughtful card in the mail, we headed to The Parks Mall to visit Vickie at Coach. (Card excerpt) *...and although I don't know you personally I would like to offer my condolences and prayers for you and your family. I just lost my grandfather* (James "Gitter" Williams) *to cancer this past Friday. My grandfather was sure to remind us that it was an attack on his body but his spirit remains untouched. Those words eased some of the hurt my family and I were experiencing and I pray it does the same for you. I wish you and your family all the best and for you to have continued strength...*That's right, this young lady was providing words for inner strength to a family she didn't even know—in *her* time of sorrow. Another person who gets it!! Life isn't all about ME.

Yours,

Frog

♦　♦　♦　♦　♦　♦　♦　♦

AUGUST 11, 2010

Dear Family,

We found ourselves back at the cancer center on Friday. Having a nice break in treatments, it was time to see if the break was going to stretch on longer or if we were headed toward serious business again. PET scan results are back and, grim-faced, the chemo doctor confirms there is cancer on the Sister's liver. The liver now takes precedence over the original tumor. The Lady continues to ask questions, but her eyes become red and watery. A fight for composure ensues. The doctor sees this as does the Sister. Chemo will start immediately on Monday, he tells us. The Lady ventures down the hall and around the corner to get a prescription filled for the Brother. She sinks into a secluded chair and prays, "God help us," as a sob escapes out loud for anyone nearby to witness.

"Are you okay?" asks Tricia, a young woman who works there.

"Yes," she answers, but it feels like a total lie.

As we head home, the Lady will continue to suppress sporadic, sharp, heavy intakes of breath that is her prelude to serious sobbing. Failing, she apologizes. Roles reverse, and it will be the Sister who becomes the strong one. Emotionally exhausted, the Lady closes the door to her temporary borrowed room, lays down, and then falls into a sleep so deep she imagines this is how it feels to be in a drug-induced coma. She'll have a nightmare whose characters consist of people who've wronged them in the past.

She wakes up shaken and feeling awful about the dream. Phone calls will go unanswered and unreturned. It crosses her mind, more than once, that she must be some sort of fake or rotten Christian to pour forth heart-felt prayers time and again, do all this fist pounding about strength, only to fall down and wallow in sadness now.

On Sunday, she puts on dud-ball clothes and plays hooky from the one place she should absolutely be—convinced she'd enter her temporary church, in her temporary life, only to be tapped on the shoulder by the deacons. *We smelled your lack of faith as soon as you entered the parking lot,* they'd say with an edge of authority. *We'll have to ask you to come with us to the pastor's office. You have some explaining to do.* This scenario would never in a million years happen; she knows this.

Family, I stopped my writing to ask the Lady if we should be writing this. She thinks for a moment then says we're not going to sugar-coat it. This is what happened and these were her feelings. She wants me to be a credible witness and in order to do that, she has to be truthful. The truth is her family is walking around with scraped knees that barely have time to form a scab before they stumble again with the next shocking bit of news. Contrary to the belief of her adult children that she's Super Woman (only not built that well), she hopes you understand she's only human. Maybe not today, no, not today, but tomorrow she'll be strong.

Yours,

Frog

P.S. The morning after we got back from traveling out of state, the Sister found one exceptionally shiny dime on her front porch. This was extremely odd because no one enters through the front door. It must have been a sign to give thanks for our safe trip home with (amazingly) no tickets or accidents.

◆ ◆ ◆ ◆ ◆ ◆ ◆ ◆

AUGUST 14, 2010

My Family!

I believe this is a landmark letter. It's hard to believe that I've been gone 111 days or 16 weeks. The Lady has been here 125 days or 18 weeks.

I've told you much about my time with this family, but there's so much more I've yet to tell. Because I write so often, and often *too* much, sometimes we all start laughing. We picture someone there coming home and asking, "Did we get anything in the mail today?" And another answering, in a really bored-to-death tone, "Just another stupid letter!" while pointing at a stack where letters are carelessly tossed on top of more letters, mostly unopened.

Have you received all my letters? I wonder if you have. I'm enclosing a white ribbon to tie on our mailbox flag to leave until you get my next letter. We'll try and find time to get over your way to check. Will you please do this for me?

Yesterday the Lady and I were at a stoplight on Cooper and Sublett when I screamed, "Oh my gosh, look! I think that's my family in front of us!"

The Lady, fighting an overwhelming need to scooch down in her seat, asks, "Are you sure?"

"No, remember I have a crummy right eye. The car *is* red. Do you see an antenna topper?"

"Oh my gosh! Yes!"

"Quick! Grab the camera!"

XO

Frog

♦　♦　♦　♦　♦　♦　♦　♦

AUGUST 18, 2010

Dear Family,

I knew even before I penned my first word, this would be my longest letter home . . .

Remember the Friday when we found out cancer had spread to the Sister's liver? We hadn't yet even made it home before the Mom called with news they'd just learned. The Dad's cancer wasn't restricted to just the removed tumor. He had a bone biopsy and they said he has multiple myeloma (bone cancer). He'll need chemotherapy and perhaps a bone marrow transplant. Silence, produced by shocked disbelief, descends. The Sister, in a voice of overwhelming compassion, face masked in sorrow, utters, "*Oh* . . . (pause), *poor Dad* . . . *It's so sad.*" Earlier that week, referring to the cancer center, "*Oh* . . . (pause) *all those poor people* . . . *It's so sad.*" Even, "*Oh* . . . (pause) *poor* (<u>orphaned-unadopted-sad faced animals-TV commercial-accompanied-with-tragic-music-playing-in-the-background</u>*)* . . . *It's so sad.*" Never once has she ever said, "*Oh* . . . (pause) *poor me* . . . *It's so sad.*"

The next day, she inconspicuously tries to disguise the broom she's carrying back to her bathroom. There's an uncomfortable edge to her voice as she passes the Lady in the hallway and confides her hair is falling out. Okay. This is it. We all knew this could happen. We just don't know the drill. Now, how it will go down? Will it be gradual—a little here, little there? Or will it be more alarming—chunks by the fist-full, clogged drains? They don't know. The Sister worries. She doesn't want to lose her hair. The whole family are big hair people. Genetics gave them more than their share. Hair irons are carried around in back pockets. Special doors are designed for their houses so big noggins clear doorways. Not really, the Lady says as she laughs, but I guess this is what makes it just a little more painful.

Monday, the sisters and I report to chemotherapy where a change of plan is disclosed. Instead of half a pouch per day, the Sister will come back every day for a full pouch. We are then herded back to conference over Tuesday's bonus treatment where she'll sit for five hours at the cancer center for another drug to drain into her port. This one's serious. It could cause ringing in the ears that could lead to permanent hearing loss and tingling of limbs to possible paralysis. *You must tell us right away if any of this happens to you,* she's instructed. We leave the center with the pump/time bomb now dispensing every 15 seconds instead of 30.

We will return Tuesday, making a conscience effort to be just "on time" instead of our usual earliness. This time, the girls ask for the room with only two chairs in it. If the Sister is going to be ill or lose her hearing and movement, privacy becomes an issue. Several pouches will drip to a suctioned out discarded emptiness before the serious pouch is produced. Relax. Lights are shut off. The door is partially shut. She breathes deeply. So far, so good. The Sister feels like eating and requests a few items that seem particularly good. The Lady jumps in her car and drives to the closest locale, 7-11, to buy the following:

- 1 package of Peanut M & M's (Sister loves)
- 1 package of Strawberry Twizzlers (Sister loves)
- 2 packages of Lays Classic Potato Chips (Sister loves and one for the Lady. What? She's hungry too!)
- 1 package of Gardettos (Sister loves)
- 1 package of mini powdered sugar donuts (Sister's very favorite and, if there's any leftovers, the Lady won't refuse if offered.)

Returning, the Lady approaches the partially shut door and gasps when she sees the Sister slumped at an awkward angle, with her mouth hanging open. *God be with us!,* the Lady's mind screams. *She's dead and the staff forgot about her with the lights out . . . all while I was out getting powdered sugar donuts and hoping for leftovers!* She rushes in and hears the Sister breathing very loudly. Setting the sack down micrometers at a time so no noise escapes, she creeps over to observe her up close. *How are we going to prevent permanent damage if she sleeps? There's no telling what kind of destruction is going on this very SECOND and we're not even aware of it!* The Lady taps the Sister's arm. Her eyes open. The Lady whispers, "Sweetheart, do you have any ringing in your ears? No? What about numbness? No? Are you sure? Okay."

(Driving home) "I don't want to lose my hair. I wish there were some way to keep the hair I have on my head."

"We could always tape it to your head with a band going around and around your forehead." (laughter)

"Then, at night I could sleep sitting up to be careful."

"Yeah, have pillows propped all around you so you don't accidentally fall over. Then we can set up a booth at the cancer center. We'll have a sign that reads: ATTENTION! Hair loss? See our booth. We've got it ALL figured out!"

Wednesday morning, the Sister is already sick even though they were told she would probably start getting sick in about three days. With a portable spit-up bag inflated, hands will be used to push back hair instead of ponytail ties, cold washcloths pressed upon her neck. We drive back to the center for the next pouch.

Thursday, the Sister will lie around with the spit-up bag in her hand while the Lady holds her hair up, in a hastily done French twist this time, as she gets sick. Hair will stick to the Lady's hands when she finally releases it. Then, back to the center where she wearily gets out of the car, spit-up bag in hand, to get a final pouch hooked up to her port. My gosh, only one more day to go. She's almost made it.

Every morning, the Lady's eyes open, she throws on her house robe, clicks on the coffee pot, finds where the Sister is lying (either on the couch or in the Sister's bedroom), and peers at her to make sure she's still breathing. The Lady says, "Hey Baby Girl. How you feelin'? I love you." Tuesday, "Hey Baby Girl. How you feelin'? I love you." And the next day and the next day, "Hey Baby Girl. How you feelin'? I love you." Friday morning arrives. The Lady says, "Hey Baby Girl. How you feelin'? I love you." The Sister says, "I love you too." But on this day her face will become devoid of emotion. For the first time ever, neither sister breaks eye contact. It goes on, and on, and on—pupils staring into pupils. Staring. Staring. Eternity! There are unspoken words to each other that they hear with their eyes. It shakes up the Lady. She told me sometimes things happen that make such an immediate impact on you emotionally, they are tattooed onto your soul to be not only remembered but forever refelt. This will be one of those times.

Friday arrives and we leave early for the cancer center. The empty pouch is ready to be disconnected. One of the staff looks at the Sister and says she doesn't look well. Since the weekend is coming up, they decide to put some more fluids in her so she'll feel better. The Sister just wants to go home. Three hours of fluid later, we leave the center with a fourth anti-nausea prescription in hand. None of the other three made the slightest difference. She hasn't kept anything down in days. Within hours of returning home, the Sister has full-blown nausea like never before. Her face starts to swell. She lies on the couch, runs to the bathroom, returns, repeats, over and over again. In the midst of this, the Lady stands at the pharmacy window as the pharmacist shakes her head, no. The pharmacist says the Sister's prescription drug coverage is maxed out for August. Three patches will be over $1,000. The Lady openly and shamelessly cries in front of her as she retrieves the prescription and leaves.

At one point, the Sister just never returns to the couch. Alarmed, the Lady goes back to the Sister's bathroom and notices the light on under the doorway from the darkened bedroom. "Baby Girl? Are you okay?" No answer. She taps softly. "Honey, are you okay?" Nothing. Getting down on the floor, she pushes the carpet back from the tile and frantically searches the one-inch view under the door, expecting to see her passed out. The floor is clear. Confused, the Lady leaves the room only to aimlessly wander around the house until she makes her way back to exactly the same one-inch empty view. The realization of what's going on makes the Lady's stomach knot. There hasn't been one time since this happened that the Lady hasn't thought of this moment and broken into immediate tears. The Sister is curled up in the closet with the door closed shut, much as you hear of animals that are wounded seeking out a quiet place to hide in their pain.

The Lady's heart breaks so hard that night when she lies down; it's a physical pain that hurts. You can walk around days, weeks, years, or *whatever*, and not even be aware your heart is in your chest, but when something hurts like this—really, really hurts—the pain is so real that you'll walk around for days feeling like you're crying inside. Huge internal sobs—even when no tears fall from your eyes. It's like a soul tattoo. The Lady won't have to search for the Sister when morning comes. She won't even have to leave her room. She'll discover her curled up asleep on the floor at the end of her bed.

On that Sunday, we find ourselves exactly where we're supposed to be.

Yours,

Frog

♦   ♦   ♦   ♦   ♦   ♦   ♦   ♦

AUGUST 24, 2010

Dear Family,

A week ago Monday, the Lady was putting on her makeup when we heard a loud commotion coming from the Sister's bathroom. It sounded like someone was kicking the cabinets really hard over and over again. The Lady rushes to the door, knocks, and foolishly asks, "Is everything okay?" The Sister says no, she's sick. This is where it gets hard for the Lady. She wants to burst through the door to be near the Sister even though there's absolutely nothing she can do. Besides, the Sister wants privacy in her pain. We learned that hard lesson by peeking under doorways.

The priority is to get our hands on some Sancuso patches—the prescription we couldn't fill. The Lady calls the manufacturer directly and starts out sounding like a professional only to end up crying to the agent, hardly able to finish her story. The agent was really nice, but rules are rules. The Lady remembers her good friend in Georgia, Lisa, is in pharmaceuticals. She sends an S.O.S. text to Lisa to see if she can get a hold of some. Who cares about the three-patch prescription? We would settle for one patch. Just get us through the week! Lisa immediately says she'll see what she can do. Who else can they call? Oh yeah, a call goes to Medicaid to ask, *Why do you have to BE like that?* One thing I've seen, it's only a matter of waiting because in every instance they've had a need it's faithfully been filled.

The other priority is to do something about the refrigerator that quit working over the weekend. Talk about when it rains! Green lunchmeat is chucked in the trash. The Lady eats a limp piece of a warm Kraft cheese slice, normally so inviting; now, all the while worrying if it can make her sick. She tells herself, if it's not green yet, she can't get sick. This is a psychological attempt to counteract the possibility she *could* get sick, but now she *won't* because that's her rule. So, lucky for her it's not going to happen!

Tuesday afternoon, the Lady answered the door and was greeted by The State of Texas Adult Protective Services. Unannounced! She introduced herself, shook the woman's hand, while pressing her other hand against her heart. Here's an instant way to be thrown back into childhood with the type of feeling you might have as you stand before the school principal! What? Are these people psychic now? What could she say? *Yeah, sure, I'll admit I felt like smacking the back of the Brother's head a few times when he was particularly ugly to me, but I DIDN'T. I want my mommy!* It turns out they were reported all right, as a family in need and they would like to buy the Sancuso prescription for us. What?

"Have you ever heard of such a thing?" the Lady asks the pharmacist at CVS, as she turns the prescription back over to her to fill.

"Never," says the pharmacist.

On good mornings, the Sister will sit at the computer and write her pen pal while the Lady sits nearby on the floor, in front of a mirror, straightening her hair. They listen to music together. Lately, they're both addicted to this one song. They play it over and over, never getting tired of it. It's called *I Would Die for You* by Mercy Me. Listen to it when you get a chance, okay?

The Lady told me everyone has to find their place in this world. She has been a wife, a mother, a homemaker; but, she has no husband, her children are grown, and this isn't her home. Such uncertainty could strangle her if she let it, yet, she's certain she's where she's supposed to be right now. This is her place in the world today. Well, I tossed and turned throughout the night thinking about her words. At sunrise I woke her and told her I was homesick. She whispered in the dark that she understood. Donning clothes and hastily tying her hair back, she brought me back to spend a moment here to watch the sun rise at my place in this world.

Yours,

Frog

P.S. The white ribbon on the mailbox flag didn't escape my notice. Thanks!

◆ ◆ ◆ ◆ ◆ ◆ ◆ ◆

AUGUST 26, 2010

Dear Family,

The new refrigerator arrived in the mail Monday in the form of a check from the siblings' Aunt Francis and Uncle Vernon in Colorado. No, they had no idea certain members of the household (okay, not "members"—just the Lady) were nibbling warm, limp cheese. The message with the enclosed check said, ". . . to use wherever it is needed most. Our Heavenly Father is in control of all that comes into our lives. He is faithful!" Boy, you can say that again! He's always faithful in providing for this family. When the Lady tells the Dad about the new fridge and the Sister's humbleness, "The boys (her sons) and I never had anything nice like that before . . . " he gets choked up and says, "I love my sisters!"

Tuesday morning, the Lady spies the Sister's unworn wig in her closet. Standing before the bathroom mirror and tucking blonde strips under the brunette wig, she's instantly transformed into their mother. She sees it clearly! Abruptly throwing open the door, she sternly says to the Sister (who's minding her own business at the computer), "If you kids don't settle down, I'm going to knock you for a loop!" They laugh hysterically.

The Sister thinks chemo has lowered her resistance and it's time to start wearing a face mask in public. She says, "But I'm too self-conscience! I can't be seen in one of those. It's too embarrassing!"

The Lady replies, "No, it's not! Who *cares*? We have to be careful; it's your health. I know! I'll wear one with you."

At the store, there are two selections in masks:

#1: Hard paper snout of an apparatus that even the Lady has serious reservations about wearing

#2: Soft pleated papered one that lays flat against face and lends an air of mystery to the wearer

Well? #2 it is!

It's early Wednesday morning when we pull into the parking lot

---

of JPS Gastroenterology. The Sister's refusing to put on her mask; no amount of discussion is going to change her mind. Discouraged, the Lady asks, "Well, you don't mind if I wear one, do you?" They laugh, but the Lady is half-serious as the more she prepared for the event the more appealing it became.

Standing beside the Sister, who is sitting on the exam table, the Lady takes two steps back to hide her face when the doctor tells them the cancer has advanced to stage four. He's signing off on her now, leaving her care to chemo and the surgeons. He then directs his eyes to the Lady who's an inch away from losing her composure. Following his line of sight, the Sister sees this and reaches over to comfort her. They both ride the elevator down in tears. *(Why'd he have to say stage four out loud? Couldn't he have just said it's bad? That hurt our feelings!)*

"Signing off just sounds like he says there's no hope!" sobs the Sister.

"NO," the Lady chokes out, correcting her (all the while wiping her face with a tissue), "that's not what he meant!"

We sit in the car for a long while, unable to get out for the next appointment. Settled in the waiting room, the Sister works on a crossword puzzle and the Lady does a word search. (*SADDLE BAG. Where is it? I can't find SADDLE BAG.*) Eyes search for an S. (*S – S – S. Sister starts with an S.*) The man sitting directly across from us intently watches her face. His eyes relay a message that says he sees what's coming. She stares at him as if to say, "You sure you want to be a testimony to this?" Grabbing a tissue in the nick of time, she buries her face and lets a couple sobs escape out loud. The Sister follows suit. Trips are made outside. Trips are made to the restroom. Neither sister is able to gain her composure. They have only but to look at each other and it's infectious.

Led to a private room to wait for the nurse, they start laughing out of control, aware everyone around can hear. The Lady says a conference will probably be scheduled for everyone involved in the Sister's care. They'll sit around a large table and the staff will likely say, "*Now, the patient seems to be doing rather well, but her sister may need medication!*" The room eventually turns silent and with that silence—a sob escapes.

What a rough day. Alone, the Lady walks through Walmart with legs of lead. All energy has evaporated. It's overcast outside. How appropriate! Driving home, she suddenly smiles when she sees the same clown on the side of the road. He always makes her smile for some reason. With headphones jammin', he dances so awesomely that she always makes a conscience effort to look for him. We pull over and walk up to him.

The Lady asks him, "Wanna take a picture? You're part of our journey. You make us smile."

Listen to this. He calls his wife on his cell phone and then hands the phone to the Lady, telling her to repeat what she'd just told him. She does. This woman, not knowing us, begins to pray this absolutely wonderful prayer for healing and strength over the phone. Our hearts are touched. Another person has been put on our path. You have just got to keep your eyes open. Pay attention!

Yours,

Frog

♦ ♦ ♦ ♦ ♦ ♦ ♦ ♦

AUGUST 30, 2010

Dear Family,

One afternoon, a nice young man walked up the driveway selling discount cards for local businesses. This family can't really use the card, but we bought one anyway to support the school. We're forwarding this to you in case you, or someone you know, can use it.

Thursday night, the Lady and I went to Legacy High School's football game in Mansfield. The Lady hasn't been to a game since 1995, and I've never been to one. We both had lots of fun watching Drew, the boy who sold us the discount card, play. He's really tough! He got right in there, knocking guys down—making us all proud.

We sat with Drew's mother and grandmother (Lisa and Amy). During half-time, we were walking to the concession stand when the Lady said, "Oh my gosh! Ladies, you are my witnesses!" as she bent down and picked a bright, shiny dime off the sidewalk. A group of teenagers were gathered nearby, and one boy said, "I thought it was supposed to be pennies." The Lady smiled and said, "Not in *our* family!" Amy said to hold a minute as she dug down in her pocket and produced a shiny dime she'd picked up off the sidewalk coming into the stadium.

Lisa's a giggler and made us forget for a moment how difficult some of the past few months have really been. The Lady, nudging her, said to look straight ahead at the moon. "Doesn't it look awesome?"

Lisa, speaking loud with authority says, "Oh! I know what that is! It's not the moon. It's MARS!" A quick perusal of the skyline by the Lady showed no other heavenly orb around so she politely mentioned she felt it was the moon. Lisa stood firm, though, saying she'd read all about it!

"Tomorrow at 12:30 in the morning, Mars will pass closer to earth than it ever will again. Only the people alive right now will ever get to observe this phenomenon and, in fact, I'm having a party at my house to see this! You wanna come?"

Well! Put like that, the Lady was now looking differently at the orb and it did, in deed, have a reddish hue that seemed very Mars-ish! Granted, she doesn't know whether Mars is red or not, since the solar system never grabbed her attention in school or beyond. However, it *must* be. I mean, there it was right there in front of her all reddish. Yes! For crying out loud! It's MARS!

Lisa's step-father, sitting behind us, having heard enough foolishness for one night, set us straight, "It's the MOON!" The Lady thought for a moment and then told Lisa, "Yeah . . . I mean, why on earth would I get up at 12:30 in the morning to look at Mars when, if this is Mars we're viewing right now, if it got any closer it'd be touching us! I'd rather see it perfectly now than stay up all night tomorrow to see it more perfectly." This set off a fit of laughter we almost couldn't recover from. Isn't life grand?

Until next time . . .

Yours,

Frog

(After this letter was mailed, it was determined that the Mars-viewing was a huge Internet hoax going around.)

♦ ♦ ♦ ♦ ♦ ♦ ♦ ♦

SEPTEMBER 1, 2010

Dear Family,

When the Brother lost his first baby during childbirth, at the time, it was the most traumatic thing that had happened to this family. That was many, many years ago, the Lady says. Moving away, it would be a long time before he'd be emotionally healthy enough to make a trip back to where his daughter was buried. On Monday, he told us he was going to go clean her grave area and pay a visit. We offered to go with him and help, but he said he needed to do this alone. He returned late in the day and said if we didn't mind, he'd take us up on the offer. It was really hot outside and his leg was giving him problems. It was back-breaking trying to paint in the etchings on the grave marker so, once again, it would allow those who passed by to know who laid there—his Jamie. The Lady and I were going to be in Cleburne anyway, on Tuesday, for her yearly physical. We said we'd swing by when we finished.

Pulling up across from Babyland, the Lady's breath catches as she sees the Brother stooped over trying to make progress on this important life mission of his. Her heart swells with pride; how hard it must be for the Brother.

Yours,

Frog

◆　◆　◆　◆　◆　◆　◆　◆

SEPTEMBER 10, 2010

Dear Family,

Where radiation is mean, chemo is that much meaner—wreaking havoc on the body—leaving destruction in its path. Annihilation of cancer cells is the goal. While innocent parties (such as the heart) sometimes take a beating in the process. Last Wednesday, the Sister was at JPS Hospital having a scan of her heart to determine if it is still up to the challenge. Is it? We haven't heard yet. At the same time, the Dad, who was in Cardiac ICU for eight days because of chemo, has a different scan of his heart. His heart says *I'm still in the fight, but I'll need some back-up.* Verbally declining the help for now, the Dad is emotionally and physically unable to face more than what he sees directly before him right now in his life and the lives of his children. Let it get just a little better. Get him back to that place where his "old self" patiently waits for him to catch up then he'll accept.

A couple years ago, the Mom gave in and purchased a cell phone for emergency purposes in case the Dad needed her while she shopped across town. Taking repeated cajoling, the Dad wanted nothing to do with one. The Lady spent a reasonable amount of time explaining the basic operation of the phone to the Mom then, periodically, took control of it to wipe out hordes of texts that kept coming through. *Can you fit me in at 3:30?* or *Highlights and shampoo tomorrow?* Clearly her phone number previously belonged to a hairdresser and, a year later, clientele were still clueless. The Mom wanted nothing to do with texting.

Earlier this year, the Dad was talked into becoming an official cell phone owner. Once again, the Lady provided a tutorial and then continued on to a *Texting 101* course. "See? It's fun because you don't spell all the words out! For = 4, I don't know = idk, because = bc, just kidding = jk." *What's this you say?* as he snatches the phone back, totally intrigued with all the coded language possibilities! He

DianaRae   61

masters it, purchases a belt holder for the phone so he's available at a moments notice. He then advances on to forwarding pictures via phone—something the Lady has shied away from learning. His children find his cell phone behavior absolutely endearing!

If ever a cell phone police were needed, citations would be issued to their sister, Donna, who sends texts after midnight not realizing the Lady sleeps with her phone next to her head as it charges. Or, Donna will call at 2 a.m. as the Lady lies totally sleep-deprived in the bed next to the Sister at the hospital. Thinking it's an emergency (I mean, look at the hour!), the Lady fumbles around in a trance to answer it. Donna, expecting to get her voicemail to leave a message, is just calling to say don't forget to ask the doctor such and such. The Lady, fighting civility says, "I love you too! Thanks for calling."

The Mom, recently wanting to get in on the action, begins producing texts left and right. Accidentally locking it in caps, not knowing how to change it back, some texts come across as shouting: YOUR FATHER AND I WENT FOR A WALK . . .

The Mom's concocted her own text language that, at times, appears in complicated Morse code. Unable to decipher the message, the Lady is then forced to break her own self-made, unofficial caregiver rule (limit calling unless really necessary) to call and ask, "Huh?" The Mom answers in half a ring while whispering, "Your father's sleeping." (*Don't you know caregiver code of ethics?*)

Don't ask them why, but for some reason, texting becomes the preferred choice of communication when you're a full-time caregiver. The following is the Lady's undeleted phone text log:

Ur mom is singin this morning. LOUD. Her heart is happy. She knows her kids will be healed. (Dad—before he was diagnosed)

Love you forever. (Mom—The Lady will never delete this one.)

Woman across room ate 3 - 4 sandwiches and a large honey bun . . . (Dad—reporting on his first day of chemo experiences)

Woke this am with Isaiah 43:2-3 When you pass through the waters, I will be with you; when you pass through the rivers, they will not sweep over you. When you walk through fire, you will not be burned; the flames will set you ablaze. For I am the lord your God...# (Mom—sends continual inspiration)

Maybe because U R beautiful! Dgs (Dad)

The Frog Letters

Say, saw where Paris got ur purse. Guess i can't afford one 4 ur bd. Maybe police auction. (Dad)

god bless my dear children with his peace know he is our stronghold # (Mom)

XO

Frog

♦　♦　♦　♦　♦　♦　♦　♦

SEPTEMBER 15, 2010

Dear Family,

In case you were wondering about the lapse between letters, it's because the Sister had chemo last week. She has treatment every day for a week. Then she has three weeks to recover before it starts again. Usually, we have a normal week or two if we're lucky, every month. Since it was a holiday week, they tried to do a five-day treatment in four days. Wednesday, she had four hours of that serious drug pumped into her port with the 24-hour pump dispensing except during that time. She made it Tuesday and Wednesday, but Thursday she woke up sick and ballooned out from swelling. The Sister sat in the waiting area for as long as she could before standing, with help from the Lady who took her arm, to make her way out to the back seat of the car to be sick in private. The Lady returned to the reception desk to let the nurses know where the Sister was. The nurses are compassionate and don't want patients being sick to this extent. Bringing the Sister back in to a private room, they pull the plug on treatment until Monday when they'll hook her back up to make up for lost time.

Friday morning, the Sister appears wearing her wig for the first time and says it's time to get used to it before next week begins. Her hair is coming out in small clumps now. The Lady overhears angry talk from the bathroom that morning as the Sister discusses her dilemma to herself while brushing her hair. People can slough the idea that it's only *hair*, but the Lady knows this truly bothers the Sister—this hair loss. Giant lint rollers are now used to capture hair off slacks, shirts, backs of chairs. A lint roller is hanging out of the Lady's purse as she transports it around with the same importance as lipstick. The vacuum bag contains a rat's nest swirled ball of hair. It feels uncanny when the Lady removes clothes from the dryer; during the cycle it's plucked stray hairs off the clothes and perfectly packaged them in compact balls for the Lady to throw away. The first time that happened, she thought about keeping one ball because to throw it away felt like a reduction in its usefulness. These small wads of hair represent something important! As the Lady showers, she'll steer the Sister's stray fallen hairs with her toe towards the drain. The act feels as reverent as a funeral procession.

The Lady didn't even know what a du-rag *was* so, weeks ago, when the Sister said she needed some, we scoured the land and ended up grabbing a variety of styles and colors at Sally's Beauty Supply. Friday night, the Sister quietly asked the Lady if she would please wear a du-rag to the cancer center next week so she didn't feel uncomfortable. "Of course!" the Lady told her; this is not an issue. Sunday, in preparation for Monday, the Lady stood before the bathroom mirror and broke open a white du-rag. It felt like a pantyhose cap and, fitting extremely snug, she thought it could become an airborne missile if it snapped off her head. As she peered into the mirror, she could hardly believe her eyes. There was little room for doubt that for some bizarre reason, with her large hair now squished down tight, her nose would be considered HUGE by most anyone's standards! With hands over both ears, she slowly started pushing the cap upward so it lifted her hair and du-rag high in the air. Oh my gosh! Now she's a Conehead! Locating the Sister in the laundry room ironing her pants, the Lady said, "Take me to your leader!" They snickered over the whole look until a split second later; the Sister burst into tears telling the Lady she knows no one else who would have willingly done this for her, and she's grateful.

An hour later, the Lady finally got the du-rag positioned where she felt "sorta cute" even though all the wrestling with her hair made it seem oily now. The Lady decided she was going to march right into the Quick Stop and gain some confidence, you know, a trial run for Monday and the crowded cancer center. Expecting one of her guy friends to be working, after they asked about the Sister (they always do), she'd ask their honest opinion. *Does this or does this NOT, in FACT, make my nose look HUGE? Be honest!* Unfortunately, some new person was at the register. Waiting for her items to be rung up, she turned to check movement behind her as a customer made his way down the aisle. He turned to make sure he'd seen right—an older white lady in a du-rag with slightly oily hair. Eyes narrowing, the Lady leaned her elbow on the counter hoping this portrayed a certain "hardness" she lacked.

XO

Frog

♦   ♦   ♦   ♦   ♦   ♦   ♦   ♦

SEPTEMBER 20, 2010

Dear Family,

Last weekend, the Lady went on her first official date since 1985. When I heard that, I said, "What? Shut up!" The Lady said, "No, really!" She wasn't much of a dater when she was young, nor is she now that she's, uh, more mature. She changed her mind a half dozen times that day. Why allow yourself to get all nervous when it can simply be avoided by just not going in the first place? However, her friends (Tom!) say, "Go! Have fun! You deserve this!"

We saw the clown last week; the Lady honked her horn as we drove past. I saw him waving his arms high over his head as if to say, *YES! I SEE you. I REMEMBER you, Frog and Lady! Have a nice day!* We both started smiling after that.

Saturday, the Lady planned to see if he (the clown) was working so she could get his wife's phone number. She told the Sister we were leaving but stalled another 30 minutes before we actually drove away. Approaching, it appeared he wasn't at work yet but, on second glance, he was in the parking lot talking to someone. This was perfect timing, His perfect timing like the dime stories, because he was talking to his wife. We were thrilled! The Lady reached her arm through the passenger window to shake her hand. This woman took, without releasing, the outstretched hand and prayed a powerful prayer for the family—for strength, for healing. The Holy Spirit surrounded us. Skeptical? I only know what I felt, and this is so.

Yours,

Frog

♦　♦　♦　♦　♦　♦　♦　♦

DianaRae

SEPTEMBER 29, 2010

Dear Family,

The Mom and Dad—partners in life for over 54 years, their love for each other has been a constant in the lives of their children. Many sentimental aspects are reminders of this bond. If you were to ask which concrete symbol attaches itself it would be doves. Did you know doves mate for life? Whenever a lone dove is spotted, a sadness drapes the hearts of this family. A collection of ceramic doves grace various spots in their home, special mementos given throughout their years together. A reminder though none was needed—of a kept promise.

Living doves have materialized recently by making appearances. You can't help but believe that, such as the shiny dimes, these are significant. Are they love signs or family connection signs? They all agree they are God-sent.

Text 08/16/10 9:35 a.m.: Dad. Something special just happened. (Brother's name) and I were sitting in the garage and a dove flew in, circled, landed on top of the door and looked at us 4 a moment. Then repeated the whole routine and flew out. Made me feel like you were here with us. I love you!

Response: Thanks for the dove story. Who knows y it showed up, may B a message 4 U or 4 me. Lv, dad

Text 08/17/10 12:27 p.m.: Dad just had my teeth cleaned at Dr. Glovers. While I was in the chair, done but waiting 4 him 2 come chk my teeth, a lone dove flew on top the column in front of my window and stayd 4 a long time. Seemed like he kept lookin rite at me.

Response: Maybe because U R beautiful! Dgs

Although the dove sightings are welcomed, they also leave behind a sense of lonely peace, if there *is* such a thing as lonely peace. The Lady would never verbalize this aloud, but it weighs on her heart that the doves, in their recent sightings, are without their mates. Is this a sign? What is the real meaning behind these visits? Is it a vision for them? Her thoughts can't help but linger a while on that concept.

Yesterday morning, the Sister opened the door from the garage into the house, pleading for the Lady to hurry. A bird was in there!

"In the house?" the Lady asked.

"No, the garage," the Sister replied.

Wondering what the big deal was, the Lady became entranced as they watched a dove walking the length of the garage on a slow stroll, checking everything out, coming extremely close to them with no fear whatsoever. He was certainly in no hurry. Eventually he left the garage as the Lady followed a few steps behind to discover its mate patiently waiting outside. Together, the two begin a leisurely walk across the neighbor's yard.

Shaking me awake, the Lady doesn't want me to miss this either. We rush across yards in our pajamas—the Lady's pink slippers becoming soaked and dirty from the grass in the process. The four of us spent quiet time in a driveway. We turn to make our way back home and the doves retrace their steps back to our garage to have another look at where we spend so much time together. Perhaps they can feel love here. This, I wouldn't doubt.

Isn't that a lovely story?

Yours,

Frog

♦ ♦ ♦ ♦ ♦ ♦ ♦ ♦

OCTOBER 5, 2010

Dear Family,

Normally, not a braggart by most standards, there are a few things the Lady simply can't prevent herself from blurting out to anyone who will listen. One is the Parents' loving relationship. Two, her kids and how awesome they truly are. Three is her Uncle Ken who discovered a gold mine, which was named after him. I mean, how cool is that? (However, she secretly fears she could go to hell for bragging on this one since it's the epitome of bragging in its rawest, totally uncalled for, form. It's just that she's so proud of him!) Finally, number four, is the impossibly low mileage she puts on her vehicles yearly.

The Lady knows there are often deadly consequences of bragging. Number four is the one that has come back to bite the Lady. No longer will she be able to point out to passengers and say, "Oh look! My odometer just rolled to _____ !" (A ridiculously low number for the age of the car)." All those random mileage polls she'd orchestrate amongst the waiting service customers at the dealership, to secretly confirm hers is still the lowest, will cease.

Her new car just had its one-year anniversary in September. It also sports over 21,000 miles. Some of these are trip-related miles but, by far, the majority of them are cancer treatment-related. Keeping the car serviced so often becomes an expense she hates, yet she can't afford to slack off on to maintain the warranty. Multiple e-mails are sent to the manufacturer letting them know she has complete comfort in the dependability of her car. She thanks them for that.

XO

Frog

♦ ♦ ♦ ♦ ♦ ♦ ♦ ♦

OCTOBER 9, 2010

Dear Family,

With all that driving, driving, driving, day-in and day-out, day, after day, after day, the Lady eventually thinks this will be her life from now on. Yes, this is it. Five years from now, there she'll be, tearing down the road taking 287 to I-20 to 820 to 287 Ft. Worth to Rosedale and the cancer center. Returning via I-35 to I-20 to 287 just to mix up the route up a bit, unless I-35 is at a standstill then they'll retrace the original route.

She becomes curious for lack of anything better to do at the moment. Exactly how many health-related appointments have they had since April? Pulling out her weekly planner, which they live by, the Lady runs a quick tally that totals 123 appointments in six months. That doesn't even count pharmacy visits. She has to draw the line somewhere because those visits would be too tedious to even count.

At some point, the Lady starts looking at housing along the way as we pass by, dreaming about how convenient it would be if we all lived happily together by the cancer center. One day, months ago, she stood outside the center and her eyes rested on a house in the distance. The house seems out of place. It sits nestled among businesses and buildings that have grown around it. Still, it's so inviting. She honestly loves it! That's all they really need, just that little house right over there in the distance. So close to the cancer center, they could walk to all the appointments. Come early evening, she pictures them sitting on the front porch laughing and reminiscing about the time before cancer dominated their lives. I imagine them missing me when I'm no longer a part of their daily lives. I believe someday they'll be a family united with not a single care in the world! Oh my gosh! What made me write that? Hmmm . . . Maybe we've all forgotten how that feels.

Yours,

Frog

◆　◆　◆　◆　◆　◆　◆　◆

OCTOBER 11, 2010

Dear Family,

It was just a good week all the way around last week! The Sister was supposed to start chemo Monday, but since she had such a tough time the last treatment, having to return the following week to complete it, they postponed her next treatment until today. That made all of us happy. Also, she managed to gain weight, getting a jump on what she loses during chemo week and the week after. The nurse and doctor were glad about that!

Shiny dimes continue to appear. Remember when we went to that football game and sat with Amy and Lisa? Amy called the Lady and said, "I'm bringing something over for you." She drove up and handed the Lady a shiny dime she'd found lying in the entryway of her house. Then, the Lady went to wash her car and right there, in "Land of Quarters," was a shiny dime in her stall. Finally, one morning last week, the Lady was in and out of the laundry room several times. Putting a load of towels in the dryer, the Sister walked past and told her there was a shiny dime in the middle of the floor. I can't see how this could have escaped our notice that many times! It's almost like it appeared for *both* sisters to see it together.

The Lady said the appearances of the dimes show He watches over us still. Since that's the case, she's recently had a really awful, awful thought that won't go away. A long time ago, someone sent a text to her. She texted back and that was the last correspondence between them. She wants them to text just one more time so she can ignore their text for a long time in retaliation. When she told me that, I said, "You've GOT to be joking!"

"Uh, yeah, sure," she said not looking me in the eye, "I mean *seriously* . . . who'd be idiot enough to admit such malicious behavior out loud?"

We've been attending the same church for six months now, but the Lady wants to scout around for others in the area. The Lady got in touch with Ken and Lu Ella. They've known her family since the

70s when they all lived in Southern California. Ken and Lu Ella have lived in this area for a long time. All those many, many years ago when the Brother lost his Jamie, Ken would come to her grave site and speak words to comfort to the family. The Lady said, "You're going to really like these people!" So we met them yesterday, in Arlington, for church.

Both Ken and Lu Ella continue to give comfort and support to the Lady. They send e-mails that make her feel strong and loved. Like this:

My dear sweet (Lady's first name), we are all weak Christians. It is in the strength of God that we are strong! You ARE strong. You just had a weak moment with your emotions. This in no way indicates that you are a weak Christian. It only shows that you are a real person and thank you for being that way with all of us. You have been a truly strong Christian and have been such an encouragement to so many people, myself included. Thank you for being so transparent with us! May the Lord lift your heart and, in some way, brighten your day today. This is my prayer! I will "up" the prayers on your behalf as well as your sister's. Sending you hugs, Lu Ella.

I had already finished this letter to you and was getting ready to mail it, but I had to add this because stuff like this keeps happening. Yesterday, the pastor's wife announced that if people have a thought that's dominating their minds that they want to be rid of, or if they have an addiction, or (several other things were mentioned), she encouraged them to come to the front. As soon as she said the part about the *thought*, I remembered what the Lady told me about the text thought so I elbowed her. She placed her hand on Lu Ella's arm and said she was going up front because this was meant for her. Whether the Lady had that awful thought or not, I can tell she feels better now and I'm glad people are placed in her path who speak to her heart.

Yours,

Frog

♦　♦　♦　♦　♦　♦　♦　♦

OCTOBER 14, 2010

Dear Family,

Monday, we were at the cancer center for five hours. It should have been a two-hour visit, but they were running behind in chemo. After the Sister's pump is connected and dispensing every 20 seconds, we leave. We stop to rent a couple movies from a Red Box, thinking she'll spend the rest of the day on the couch; instead, she asked the Lady if she felt like walking. We drove over to the lovely park off Curry. Have you been there? Getting out of the car, they begin a fast-paced walk around the trail. The Sister tells the Lady that every step she takes is building her body up. It may even make her live a day longer; you never know! After the second lap together, the Lady sits on a bench and watches the Sister across the horizon taking a final solo walk. Watching every step taken, far off in the distance, she distinguishes the chemo pump strapped to the Sister's waist and recalls the words she spoke earlier about living another day. She draws near, passes us by, as we continue to watch her retreating form as she leaves us again. The Lady's eyes fill to over-flowing with tears of love, hope, and sadness. The sadness, realizing so many years have passed them by and, try as she desperately does, she fails to recall a single time they have taken a walk together. The thought of such wasted time makes her sick.

Tuesday was the day for that awful five-hour extra drug they give the Sister. Instead of going straight home, she surprised us and wanted to walk in the park again. Hoping she gains some strength, maybe another day to live, the Lady gladly turns in that direction. We all know it's only a matter of time before the drug takes effect and she won't be able to make this walk for a while.

Wednesday, the Lady wakes up assailed by a wave of nausea that she's sure is strictly nerve-related. She's concerned not knowing if the Sister is ill this morning or, worse, ill while she slept right through it. The cancer center is behind schedule causing the three of us to sit for six hours when normally it would have been two. This isn't normal. It's not just difficult on us but also for every person in the packed waiting room. In three days, we've spent 16 ½ hours just within the walls of the center. This day, the Sister does not walk the trail. Having not eaten all day, she's nauseated and chills invade her body. Refusing food, she lies on the couch with two heating pads and a blanket for warmth. Asleep within minutes, she sleeps deeply for several hours. In the early evening, she wakes for a moment and makes her way to the restroom, using the walls for support. The Lady notices this and begins her vigil over her, starting now, by closely following her back to the couch.

The smell of brewed decaf permeates the air. "Is it still the same day?" the Sister asks, hoping morning has come and she's already made it through the night.

"Yes honey (sigh), it's still the same day . . . " the Lady answers.

Yours,

Frog

◆ ◆ ◆ ◆ ◆ ◆ ◆ ◆

OCTOBER 19, 2010

Dear Family,

The actions of one of the siblings would produce a domino effect on the rest of the family. Most of them begin to contemplate, discussing among themselves and their adult children, arrangements for their final resting place. One may feel the action is morbid and a sign of giving up—not so for this group. Remember long ago when I told you members of this family were preparers? They prepare now, knowing their time here on earth is but a temporary journey. Staying here forever has never been the real goal nor an option. We are none invincible. I realize for the very first time this includes me.

The Parents wish to return to their roots in Rifle, Colorado. This is the land of their childhood as well as their children's. Each carries a piece of the family homestead in their heart. Memories abound here—generations of them. Time could never remove the connection they feel to this one spot in the world. The Parents choose the old cemetery that sits high on a bluff above town. The Dad's parents and grandparents rest here. The Mom's great-grandmother and grandparents are here too. Aunts and uncles from both sides, as well. The Parents suppose, when the time comes, they'll rest near them.

The Lady asks the Brother what he wants to do. *Wanna join mom and dad in Rifle?* He's one of the ones who finds it rather doomsdayer-ish. The Lady, herself, decides not to make a decision right now about where her final resting place will be.

Initially, the Sister voices she wants to be near the Dad, placed next to him if nobody minds. The two share a bond between them that erases the miles that actually separate them. Changing her mind, torn, the Sister's strongest roots are here in Texas. Her children live here. Together, the Sister and Lady walk the length of a nearby cemetery. It's a beautiful day. The Sister stops under the canopy of a large Texas scrub oak. A nice breeze ruffles their hair. She points to a spot, this one right here. The choice is made; with that decision, it feels surreal knowing this is where she'll be waiting.

An unexpected monetary gift arrives from their Uncle Stan and Aunt Louise who live in Oregon. Another arrives the following week from their Uncle Jim in Colorado. The Lady meets with the woman who manages the nearby cemetery, a few days later. She tells us her family's been a part of maintaining the cemetery for a long while. Her father, for the longest time, was the caretaker. He's now buried in the upper part of the cemetery along with her mother. Her brother wants to rest near them. Sweeping her arm across the landscape, she says various cousins have chosen spots in the lower section. As the two of them walk the grounds, they stop to spend a moment staring at the marker where her daughter lays—a victim of cancer four years earlier. She tells the Lady her daughter was a happy person, always laughing. Perhaps in some way, the woman hopes by telling another, the daughter will continue to be remembered. She's telling the right person. The Lady *will* remember because when she peers down at the marker, it takes her breath. Her daughter's first name is eerily close to the Sister's first name, and her middle name is two letters off from being the Lady's middle name.

Déjà vu feelings sweep over the Lady. It's another beautiful day. The breeze has returned. Maybe it's a constant; time will tell. Slowly making her way toward a certain tree, however did she think she was strong enough to do this? Coming to a stop, the Lady points with her toe to the Sister's spot under the oak.

Voice catching, "This one . . . right here," she tells the woman. The choice is made.

Yours,

Frog

♦ ♦ ♦ ♦ ♦ ♦ ♦ ♦

OCTOBER 22, 2010

Dear Family,

Sunday before last, a Sancuso patch was placed on the upper arm of the Sister in preparation for chemo treatment all week. At the end of August, we were told if the patch didn't control her severe nausea, well, it's just the final resort. None of her chemo treatments could be considered anything other than living nightmares. Hope is placed in the patch to *some* extent but, making a conscience effort, the sisters change up their routine drive to the cancer center. This time, prayers are issued out loud as the center draws near. Since nobody said prayers have to always be so formal with bowed heads, they opt for a more personal approach. The Lady also decides, during Monday's prayer and the remaining prayers that week, to go ahead and ask that He make this an easy week for the Sister, that the drugs work to her benefit and, if it's His will, they'd appreciate it if she weren't so sick. It's really hard to pray for these things even though scripture says otherwise. They don't want to come off as overly greedy in their requests.

On Thursday, the Sister mentions that she can't believe she is not sicker than she is. Other Thursdays bore chaotic effects by now. "It must be the new prayers," she says. The Lady has to agree. Me too! Sure, the Sister is still sick. Chemo drugs are harsh chemicals racing through the body, causing everything internal to burn like fire, especially the digestive tract. Extremely painful mouth sores appear. This time her tongue swells. Her liver lets her know, by way of sharp pains, it's not happy with whatever is filtering through it. *You're being healed*, they tell it!

With the Sister's nausea under control, what could have been considered the most horrific thing that could happen after chemo week, the thing we've always secretly fretted over, becomes an inconvenience and not the end of it all. Saturday, the Lady woke up feeling like she may be getting sick. (Unknown at the time, she'd get really sick and bedridden for days with a sinus infection.) Anyway, on this day she drove down to the home where she lived for 13 years.

Walking into her former residence after being away for so long, her very first thought is, *Man! I'm a great decorator!* She walked to the back bedroom and kissed her 22-year-old son from a distance in case she's contagious. Eventually, walking into his restroom to wash her hands, her eyes are drawn to the tile under the cabinets. A shiny dime laid there. Hmmm . . . This is an oddly normal occurrence now! She picks up the dime and pockets it. Breathing a sigh of thankfulness, she needed this one.

Yours,

Frog

♦ ♦ ♦ ♦ ♦ ♦ ♦ ♦

OCTOBER 26, 2010

Dear Family,

Honoring the Sister's request, the Lady dons her du-rag for chemo week. She also does this in support of every cancer patient taking on the fight of all fights to live. The Lady realizes there's a good chance chemo treatments will end next month. She feels this is so. She learned early on, the scarf-tied du-rag is much easier to put in place, but it's only bearable for about six straight hours at a time. Ripping it off her head one day, after an especially back-logged chemo day, she apologized to the Sister and spent several minutes fingering her headache. Whereas, the snug panty hose-type du-rag that threatens to snap off and become air-borne, it's nothing short of dangerous! Best not to wear these if there's any possibility it'll need to be removed before returning home; the bands are so tight they leave a deep crevice of a ring around the wearer's forehead. Not only do you look weird in public with the forehead indention visible, your hair is also smashed beyond repair. The Lady said it *did* seem like she stood out more too but, then again, she could be totally paranoid over nothing!

Yours,

Frog

♦ ♦ ♦ ♦ ♦ ♦ ♦ ♦

OCTOBER 28, 2010

Dear Family,

It's a long standing joke here. Remember when I first came here all those months ago? At the time, the Lady was taking the Brother to radiation every day. On those days, she would be trying to get treatment started for the Sister. She's been a fixture in the cancer center since then. What's so funny is, since so many people see her so often, they assume she must have cancer. It certainly doesn't help matters that the Lady wears a du-rag which, unintentionally, stereotypes her and confuses people.

One day, before the Sister had begun her treatments, she went with the Brother and Lady to the center. The Lady went to the chemo physician's window to ask several questions that pertained to the Sister. She was asked to take a seat. Eventually, the nurse came out to find us. When she approached, both sisters stood up. The nurse began relaying information to the Lady. The Sister politely interrupted to say, "I'm the one with cancer." The nurse looked at her for a split second then continued directing all her conversation to the Lady, as if to say, *Yeah, you and everyone else here, but this is the patient I'm talking to . . .* The sisters still laugh about that day, but it kind of gave the Lady the creeps. She went home and studied her face in the mirror to see if perhaps the nurse saw something in her that says she has cancer. I mean, the odds are high in this family, right?

Another time, the Lady was leaning toward the chemo physician's window talking to the women behind the glass when the Sister poked her head behind the Lady's shoulder to have a look. Everyone was surprised. They said, "So *this* is what the patient looks like!" However, yesterday was the best of the best! The Sister had an appointment with her chemo doctor, Dr. Choufani, to see how she's recovering from her last treatment. The sisters and I were led into a room and the nurse asked if we were cold because, if we were, there were blankets in the second drawer. The Lady *was* cold so she grabbed a blanket then sat in her usual chair as the Sister climbed up on the exam table. While waiting for the doctor, we were laughing at the stories I just told you about. Then the Lady said we should test Dr. Choufani to see if he really knows who the patient is. The Sister got up and sat in the chair beside me and the Lady, wrapped in a blanket, climbed up on the table. She leaned her head back with a forlorn look on her face. We really hooted over that. Oh my gosh, it was hilarious!

Normally, without fail, the doctor will walk in and shake all our hands, then he'll turn to the Sister and say, *How are you feeling today?* The Lady was excited about being asked this because she planned to tell him she had a hacking cough because of a sinus infection that moved down into her lungs. How'd he plan to treat her for that, she'd ask. Soon after, Dr. Choufani walked into the room. He looked at the Sister, then over to the Lady, then over to me. A huge smile appeared on his face. He knew *exactly* who his patient was and thought we were funny for trying to pull a joke on him.

Yours,

Frog

♦ ♦ ♦ ♦ ♦ ♦ ♦ ♦

OCTOBER 31, 2010

Dear Family,

As of today, I've been gone 189 days—about 27 weeks. The Lady has been here for 203 days or 29 weeks. For over six months, I've been away from you. I imagine you're missing me as I'm missing you. Remember, if you ever need me to come home, just tie that yellow ribbon on the mailbox flag. Every now and then, we drive by and check. I promised you long ago I would be home someday; I'm just not ready right now. We're constantly going places, meeting people, and seeing things. Besides, I can't leave this family until I know the end of their story. I think you understand this and also wait to see what becomes of them.

Last night, the Lady and I were invited to go with a friend to a costume party at someone's house. Even though we didn't know anyone else at that party, we had a nice time. The Lady's making me dress up like a baby for Halloween. I don't appreciate that! I wanted something more manly, but we couldn't find anything at the costume shop in my size.

We're also sending you a gift card for two dozen cookies from the mall cookie store. It's time to spread some joy. A dozen are for you, but the second dozen is for someone you know who's going through a difficult time. So, think carefully and go brighten his or her day.

Yours,

Frog

♦ ♦ ♦ ♦ ♦ ♦ ♦ ♦

DianaRae

NOVEMBER 4, 2010

Dear Family,

The Brother has been cleared to drive again. Since the second skin graft, his right leg has healed nicely. It's no longer a horrible-looking open wound. He's back out in the world. He travels by bus, by plane, and then he travels by car. He misses his daughter and journeys far to see her. The Brother stays gone for weeks this time. Returning with a limp, he no longer walks with his cane. He shows the Lady his hip where a mysteriously huge water blister, the size of his fist, has formed and burst open. It's alarming in size. Even more alarming is the reason it would even appear. What next? What now?

The Lady quizzes the Brother, "Were you bedridden while away and lying around for hours on your hip?"

"No, I don't know how it happened," he says.

The Lady insists he go see a doctor. She's afraid more is going on with the Brother than they know. A shell of his former self, he's about the thinnest we've ever seen him. Still tube-fed, he often talks about when the day will come when he can eat a cheeseburger.

We don't know what he searches for out in the world, but he comes back lost. He doesn't search in the right place. We can't help him to be happy. The Lady tells him the world will let you down, people will let you down, but the only one who will never let you down is Christ.

His PET scan is finally scheduled to see if he's cancer-free. The following week, the results are in. The body is all clear except for his head. Red warning lights say something is going on and needs to be checked. Tuesday, the Brother and Lady are back on the second floor of JPS Hospital. Let me tell you about the second floor. It's nothing like any doctor's office you'll ever visit. When you exit the elevator, chairs are tightly lined up side by side in a square around nearly the entire floor. On most any given day, the place is packed. We walk a complete square out of curiosity and it takes 225 normal steps to complete the square. There are 50 rooms numbered around the square's interior. Nurses will open random doors and yell, *So and so to room 26 . . .* or whatever room. On the other side of the rooms, the very interior of the floor, are the office cubicles of nurses, doctors, and staff.

This day, the Brother's surgeon looks in his mouth and says he doesn't like what he sees. Shining a light into the recesses, he asks the Lady if she'd like to have a look. Well, no she doesn't *want* to have a look but, before she has time to respond, she's leaning down and looking into the Brother's mouth. What does it look like? It looks all wrong is what it looks like. You see normal mouth tissue everywhere until you get to the area where the jaw hinges and then, well, it's just bad.

The surgeon asks the Brother if he is right-handed; he is. He then lifts the sleeve covering the left arm and studies it while saying not to let blood or anything else be drawn from that arm; they may need to use the skin. The Lady feels ill. Of course it only makes sense that they can't use his other leg this time or he would be crippled. How much more? What will he lose this time? There are so many questions that just can't be answered now.

It's a cold, rainy day. How appropriate, once again, the weather cooperates with the mood. Driving home in a downpour, the Lady thinks she may pass out after remembering the problems the Sister told her about. The problems she wasn't around to witness when the Brother first got home from his major surgery in February. The tracheotomy was the worst. Once he was home, the tube separated while they were cleaning it and panic ensued. What to do? What to do? Gosh! Will he have one of those again and can she bear to put it back in place if that happens again? Well, she'll *have* to, but why can't home health care staff just spend the night at a patient's home for a while until everyone's comfortable with the situation? Someone needs to get right on that idea! Soon!

Day surgery is scheduled a week away. A second in-hospital stay surgery is scheduled for the week after that. Their poor Parents— when they find out, it's going to be skinned knees again. The Lady sends the Mom a text: *I can do ALL things through Him who gives us strength.* (Philippians 4:30) *Say it out loud.* She finds that saying Scripture out loud is so much more empowering than keeping it inside. Surprisingly, the Brother takes the news well. He hopes this time he comes out with a working jaw so he can eat.

Returning home, the Lady climbs into bed and pulls the covers up to her ears. Lying on her side, she remembers she hates lying on her side with makeup on; it crunches up your eyelashes and leaves them unruly when mascara-coated. Yet, she remains unmoving. Looking at her cell phone, on the other side of the bed, she thinks maybe she should call Lu Ella. Her arm never reappears from under the covers to complete the task because it's cold in the house. As if reading her mind, the Sister appears and asks if she's cold because she's turning the heater on for the first time. "It's going to make that burnt smell," she says.

The Lady's mind drifts to her most recent nightmare. Someone is chasing her one night through an unknown building. She almost runs into a young girl. Looking at each other, face to face, both are pleasantly surprised to see the other. The Lady only has seconds to speak with her and tell her the most important thing she can.

"I love you. Your mom loves you. There's never been a day she hasn't thought of you."

"Is this true?"

"Yes!"

The Lady takes off running. Losing her footing in flight, her hands touch the floor as she regains her balance.

The young girl remains in the exact position, as if she were a statue, then turns her head to the left to watch the Lady's retreat. Coming to an abrupt halt, the Lady realizes she's in a high tower under construction, a skyscraper that's little more than large steel beams of framework. Deathly afraid of heights, yet frantic to escape, she gets down on her hands and knees and begins to cross a long steel beam. The wind whips up in a mad fury around her.

Yours,

Frog

♦ ♦ ♦ ♦ ♦ ♦ ♦ ♦

NOVEMBER 6, 2010

Dear Family,

"I'm just sick to *death* paying $19.95 for cheap reading glasses and then losing them," the Lady tells our neighbor, Amy, one day. Amy says she used to have the same problem, but found it easier to buy a bunch of them from a dollar store. She has them lying in various spots throughout her house now.

A few days later, the Lady lost her glasses *again*. Feeling rather lazy, she called Amy to see if she could borrow a pair until the following day when she had full intention of taking Amy's advice and buying several.

Being thoughtful, Amy shows up with a store sack filled with new glasses, one of each prescription offered. The Lady takes the one she knows is probably her prescription. It's a practical pair and she claims them as her own. Then she picks up a bold pink pair that seems like someone much younger would wear. They're almost toyish-looking and would certainly attribute a certain level of immaturity to the wearer. She must have these! Holding them in the air, she tells Amy she loves them.

The ear piece on the practical set snapped off within days. Now the Lady had every excuse to wear the pink ones. One day, the sisters and I took off to CVS pharmacy. When we got home, the pink glasses were missing. The Lady tore her purse apart and rummaged all through the car. With her cell phone poised in hand, waving the store receipt in front of the nephew's face, she asks him to hurry up and call out the CVS phone number. She can't read it. Time is of the essence! It's imperative she call right away before they're stolen! The clerk answers, has a look around the Reece's cup display where the Lady said to pay particular attention, and says they aren't there. The Lady knows they have to be there. She *knows* it! The clerk scribbles down her phone number so he can call the very minute they're located.

The next morning, the Lady, nephew, and I were going to the

post office when the Lady tells us she's *got* to stop at CVS. She just knows her glasses are there. She can't quit thinking about them. As we approached the same parking space as the day before, she could see them lying trampled to pieces. Her heart stopped. Oh yes, she knows *exactly* what must have happened. As we were walking back to the car, she stopped and hastily unwrapped her special Halloween pumpkin-shaped Reese's Cup before getting into the car. The sound of her glasses falling off the side of her purse must've been muffled by the deliciously over-powering sounds of a Reese's Cup being unwrapped. . .

Yours,

Frog

♦ ♦ ♦ ♦ ♦ ♦ ♦ ♦

NOVEMBER 10, 2010

Dear Family,

It's du-rag week again and it arrived faster than any of us would have liked, especially for the Sister. Sunday, she voices aloud her body is just not ready; she can tell. She should ask them to delay treatment another week. Silence meets that statement as all of us who gather in that room know, sure as the sun will rise and the Lady will pour too much cinnamon vanilla creamer into our coffee, come tomorrow the Sister will be hooked back up to the pump regardless of wishful thinking today.

Early morning Tuesday, the Brother, Lady, and I made our way to JPS Hospital Out-Patient Center. For the Brother, it's biopsy and testing day in preparation of surgery next week. Leaving him, we walk across the street to the main hospital to have the Sister's prescriptions filled. This process takes a couple of hours on a good day and four hours on a bad day. We sit in the dark, number five in line, before the staff even arrives. This will be a good day.

Knowing somewhere in the building is a cafeteria we've never found, we opt to complete unfinished business at the McDonald's in the hospital. Ordering breakfast, the Lady says, "Back in May, my sister was hospitalized for eight days here. One day I ordered $10.57 worth of food. The next day, I noticed a sign here saying debit cards were not being accepted. That transaction never cleared my bank. Can you add $10.57 to my order today?" The server left for a moment then returned and handed us a card for a free Value Meal.

The server said, "The manager asked that I give this to you and tell you, you're the last honest person in the world today. Thank you!"

We ran into our friend, Raymond, who works at the main hospital. We met him back in May. She was a random stranger entering the building when he said to the Lady, "How are you doing today?"

"Fine!" she replied in a cheerful tone.

Hours later, while leaving the building in tears, distraught over the Sister, we ran into him again. He asked if everything was okay and we could tell the question was not a generic one; he genuinely wanted to know. Anyway, all these months later, we see Raymond all the time. Now when we arrive, he says, "Princess!" when he sees the Lady. Sometime in reply, she rummages in her purse and squirts cucumber melon spray mist into the air. It's their routine, odd as it is; we've all come to expect it. He's such an inspiration not just to us, but to a whole lot of people there. Definitely a part of our journey.

Today was also the long five-hour treatment day for the Sister. Driving the Brother home then turning around for the cancer center, it will be a long day for us. The Lady eats too many Lorna Doone cookies while waiting around. She's seriously considering writing to the company to commend them on their product. However, right now, she feels too sick to bother since she's eaten so many. Drinking juice with them, she hopes this completes the whole meal where she can now label it sort of nutritious.

Late in the day, we went outside and sat on the sidewalk curb so I could write you this letter as we waited. An older gentleman asked the Lady if she was also waiting for a ride. She nodded her head no. He asked, "You don't have this crud too, do you?"

"No, my brother, sister, and dad have it." Noticing he's wearing a patient bracelet, "What kind do you have?"

"Myeloma," he replies. It's the same cancer the Dad has. "But they stopped treatment on me. Oh! Here's my ride." A medical transport taxi pulls up and the gentleman gets in, shuts the door, and brake lights are released.

Oh my gosh! It's now or never! The Lady bolts from the sidewalk, rushes to the taxi door, and pulls it open. "I apologize. I'm sorry," she says, while casting a glance up at the driver then back to the gentleman. "I have to know—why'd they stop treatment?"

He looks at the Lady and his face becomes masked in confusion. "I don't know why," he says in a voice that's part whisper. They look at each other for a few moments before she shuts the door. Walking tiredly back to the concrete curb, she sits back down and continues thinking about the man.

Yours,

Frog

◆ ◆ ◆ ◆ ◆ ◆ ◆ ◆

The Frog Letters

NOVEMBER 16, 2010

Dear Family,

It's 5:30 a.m., and the three of us sit at JPS in anticipation of what will happen today for the Brother. The biopsy results came back clear. The surgeon wants it retaken to try and find out exactly what is going on with his mouth. We're not even sure he will have surgery today even though they've allotted him six hours in the operating room. Here we are. Here we sit and wait, something at which we are quite experienced. In the meantime, I will try to tell you what it's like to live the life of a caregiver from what I've seen.

I already told you about all the driving we do with hours and hours of waiting and sitting for one thing or another. Right now, it's 7:37 a.m. The Lady and I blew some time with breakfast at the hospital McDonald's, looking around for Raymond, and chatting in the waiting room with a fellow wait-er. We were just told the Brother is now in surgery. That probably means the biopsy procedure has begun.

The Lady plays the role of secretary. Paperwork is completed for siblings. Trips are made to Staples to run copies. The schedule book is kept in tip-top shape with phone calls placed to rearrange appointments that clash between patients. There is more waiting. Being stuck on hold is common. Maneuvering automated phone systems, as well as trying to crack the code to reach a human to answer billing questions is a challenge. The Lady makes post office trips to keep stamps in supply to mail my letters home. Correspondence on behalf of all is completed. Thank you cards are written in a timely manner. She stays on top of it so it never becomes overwhelming. I mean, no telling what tomorrow brings.

She's the house-maintainer. A clean family already, the weekend before chemo treatments is spent doing a shakedown thorough scouring. Details aren't overlooked. Doorknobs are even sanitized. Laundry is never neglected. Nightly, she places a clean towel out for the Sister and places her wig back on its stand. Yard work is done as frequently as time allows. Pansies are planted and mulch is spread this week. Reading over my shoulder, she just told me not to bring up the backyard as she'll get to it this weekend.

Training the household early on, she placed a notepad on the counter next to the phone. Telling the family if we're running low on anything, to write it down. Sunday morning, after dressing for church, she'll take the notepad and rewrite the list, organizing it in order of the aisles of Walmart so there's no backtracking. After a quick perusal, pantry and refrigerator shortages are added to the list because the minute we leave church, you'll find us stocking up. Random, frivolous items are placed in the cart for the Sister. (*Here! Individual packaged marble jack cheese blocks. For YOU. Sure, the larger block was cheaper, but these are cute and easy to open. See? I got these because I love you and want you to have a good life.*) These gestures are noticed.

Also, the Lady is the comedian/entertainer, inadvertently and sometimes intentionally, making everyone laugh. This comes naturally for her ever since they were children. Hey! I, too, do this through my letters home that I sometimes let them read.

The Lady is a spiritual supporter. Placing one hand on the knee of a passenger and one on the steering wheel, prayers are offered up. Praise music plays from KLTY or she'll put in the Third Day or Kari Jobe CDs and play the Sister's favorite songs. I noticed if the Sister's feeling well she'll say, "Play it again!" If she's sick, the Lady will ask, "Wanna hear it again?" The Sister replies in a tired voice, "If you want . . . " It doesn't feel the same.

One night, a couple weeks ago, the Lady and I went to lay down and she started to pray. Right away, a calmness came over us and words were placed on her heart. Getting out of bed, we walked through the darkened house to where the Sister laid. Kneeling beside her, the Lady took her hand, "I was just praying and I felt God wanted me to tell you that He knows who you *are* and He's with you and walking beside you. Whatever happens, it's His will and you're going to be okay."

The Lady got an e-mail earlier that same day from Linda. (Lu Ella introduced us at church.) The e-mail said they were having a healing service the next morning at church; Marilyn Hickey was leading it. I didn't know who she was, but she's is a well-known Christian speaker who travels the world. The Sister was too sick to go, so the Lady and I told her we would go and stand in her place. Instead of saying our names when we prayed, we said the Sister's name out loud.

It's almost 9:21 a.m. We sit for a while next to the Brother. He's in recovery with a blue hair net on his head and doesn't even know we're here. The Lady asks the nurse questions. *At least he didn't have the* . . . (the nurse scans his chart*) radical neck resection he was scheduled for.* It takes everything for the Lady not to ask if that would've involved him coming home with a trache tube. We won't find out what happens next until next Tuesday, when we visit the surgeon. Another week. This feels like a good thing for some reason. The three of us will be home before noon.

Finally, the Lady is also a mother to her siblings. She tries to comfort them, offer security, normalcy, and sometimes scolds. Lighting a cinnamon-apple scented candle to burn, she's a homemaker. Her devotion to the greater good knows no bounds. There simply aren't any. After treatments, she'll pull the car into Albertson's and make mad dashes through their wonderful produce aisles if the Sister mentions an orange sounds good. Or, remembering how the Sister loves Olive Garden's salad dressing, the Lady will burn a trail across town and back to produce these offerings of love.

Yours,

Frog

♦ ♦ ♦ ♦ ♦ ♦ ♦ ♦

NOVEMBER 23, 2010

Dear Family,

I'm sorry I couldn't find the time to write sooner. Last week was nuts. I already told you about Tuesday and the Brother's second biopsy. Later, the Mom told us their Grandmother took a serious fall, landing on her face. She broke her nose and wrist. They suspect bleeding on the brain. She and the Lady are close. I met her when we visited the Mom and Dad in North Carolina. The Lady was so upset hearing this, we drove home in a rush to look at the appointment book to see if we had time to get there and back, but we don't. One thing on the Lady's Bucket List is to be with her Grandmother in her final hours.

When the Grandmother first arrived in the emergency room by ambulance, she began mumbling then raised both arms in the air toward heaven (even her broken one). She said, "He loves me. He loves ME. He LOVES me!" Then she fell into a coma for two days. The Dad, after visiting, said her broken hand was black. Her lips were bruised. She looked like she was in a car accident. She woke up to the sound of the Dad's voice the next day. "I thought I was in the rapture!" she said. Intrigued, the Lady asked the Mom to pry for details. What did she see? How did she feel? What'd she think? The Mom questioned her then asked, "Did you see Jesus?" Anxiously awaiting any revelation the Grandmother could shed on her experience, it turned comical when she couldn't recall anything whatsoever. Jesus? No, she didn't see Him but she *was* convinced, wherever she was, the rapture was taking place. Well, certainly for us, we're glad the rapture wasn't taking place because we're still here! The rest of the week, her health was a yo-yo. She's recovering. She's not going to recover. Back and forth. The uncertainty of the situation prompts the Lady to sit down and write her Grandmother a heart-felt letter. She tells her every single thing she'd tell her if they were face-to-face.

A CT Scan is ordered for the Sister before any more chemo is given. This will let the doctor know if her body is responding to treatment. She's had other CT scans, but this one is different. She is given two tall bottles of banana-flavored stuff to drink within two hours. The Lady knocks on the radiation window with the intent of asking if the Sister has to wait an hour before starting the second bottle. Instead, she says, "She wants to know if she can have a third bottle." Everyone laughs because no one asks for *more*. Finishing both bottles, the Sister leaves to have scans taken then reopens the door and waves at us to come with her.

The CT technologist, with over 20 years experience, shows us a trip through the Sister's body on a screen. It's fascinating! She scrolls around and names all the Sister's organs and says, "Here's the liver. You have to have your liver to live. That's why it's called the *live-er*." Well, call us doh-doh heads, but it never dawned on us that's how the liver got its name! They can take any part of this scan and chop it, chop it, chop it down to micrometers of the area they want to examine. She's not allowed to tell us any type of diagnosis or what her thoughts are when she views the Sister's liver and tumors, but she pulls up a scan taken back in April. This scan shows a healthier looking liver than the scan of her liver in June. Zooming in on the April scan, the technologist positions the scan so it matches the same shot of the liver scan for today. Showing us before and after pictures, side by side, I have to tell you, spots that were there in April are gone. A larger spot is now hardly there. We got in the car and the Lady said, "Thank you, JESUS!"

The Sister went to sweep the driveway and found a shiny dime lying there. The Dad walked out of the bank, almost to his car, and found his shiny dime. The Lady crawled in the passenger seat of her son's car and the tip of a shiny dime was peeking from underneath the floor mat.

"It's probably mine," he says, as she holds it up.

"Nope, this one's mine," she tells him while slipping it in her purse, "from heaven."

Yours,

Frog

◆　◆　◆　◆　◆　◆　◆　◆

NOVEMBER 26, 2010

Dear Family,

Yesterday was Thanksgiving so I decided to make a list of what I'm thankful for:

I'm thankful for the family here who's embraced me and let me be a part of their journey.

I'm thankful for shiny dimes!

I'm thankful for the cancer center, JPS Hospital, and all the patients, doctors, and nurses I've met. I'm thankful for the way they're trying to help the Brother and Sister get well.

I'm thankful to God for helping the doctors make wise decisions about their care. Tuesday we found out the Brother's biopsy results are probable first stage carcinoma, but they want to wait a month to do a third biopsy instead of a radical neck resection on a "probable." Wednesday, we found out the Sister's original tumor has shrunk almost 80 percent!

I'm thankful the Lady's car runs well so we never get stuck anywhere.

I'm thankful for the hundreds and hundreds of people who know me now and send me notes of support through the Lady. (I'm not bragging, but you wouldn't believe how popular I'm getting!)

I'm especially thankful when chemo weeks are over. I'm definitely thankful for that!

I'm thankful I haven't lost my right eye.

For the times we drive by the house, I'm really thankful (more than I can tell you) for you, my family. I'm thankful you've allowed me to stay gone far longer than I ever thought I would be. I'm also thankful you continue to take care of, and hold for me in my absence, my rightful place in this world.

XO
Frog

♦ ♦ ♦ ♦ ♦ ♦ ♦ ♦

Dear Family,

After church on Sunday, we took Donna to the airport so she could get back to New Jersey. If you're wondering if a shiny dime incident occurred, since she's the original dime story teller, it *did*. Saturday, the Lady smoothed clean sheets on a mattress in her room, in preparation for Donna to stay with us instead of the hotel where she'd been staying. For half the night, the three of us chatted and lounged in there as the Lady worked crosswords and Donna read my copy of my letters home to you. (Yeah, I'm just vain enough I like to reread my stuff sometimes!) I hounded her to reveal which part she was laughing at. *Wasn't I funny?* Or, I would push a tissue toward her if I remembered a particularly sad letter was coming up. Reading for a while, chatting between letters, we'd leave to snack on Thanksgiving leftovers, come back, and repeat the process. At one point, Donna went into the Sister's room to grab a blanket then came back and got comfortable again on her mattress. With all the up/down activity from leaving and coming back so many times, at one point she rustled the blanket back into place and a shiny dime bounced up in the air and landed on the blanket. I love that happened with both those sisters together this time.

One Sunday, the pastor was giving the sermon and said some people walk around complaining about all the bad things that happen to them and how the devil was responsible. However, he reminded us that God sees our actions and He does punish. Sometimes those bad things that happen are just a good old-fashioned spanking from Him. The Lady thought about the Brother. Sometimes, he is crotchety. No one wants to endure what he's had to; we all understand this and sympathize with his circumstance. However, for the past two weeks he's been sleeping his life away on the couch. A blanket is pulled up to his head and his back is to us. He did rouse himself while Donna was here, but she caught a glimpse of the other side of him when he *is* awake. Before she arrived, he'd gotten in the habit of slamming doors and not talking.

One night, as the Sister laid on the couch recovering from chemo and quietly talking to the Lady, he slammed out to the garage again. The Sister got a distraught look on her face. She worries about him and worrying isn't good for her health. The Lady got up, went out to the garage, and asked him if there was some particular reason he felt it was necessary to slam the door. He stood up, walked up to the Lady (settling in an intimidating stance), and yelled he *didn't* slam the door, but if she *wanted* him to, he'd show her what slamming the door was! Well, at first the Lady looked at him, sizing him up, and thought, *He's taller, but I think I can take him down. . .* Arguing ensued that can only be recognized as fairly normal between siblings in their teens! That's right! They were reduced to childish behavior. Shame on them. I'm telling you this story so you know nothing of this world is ever perfect, certainly not the Lady. Sometimes, I fear I've led you to believe otherwise. Life is difficult. The journey is rough. We all make mistakes.

Donna mentions, between letter reading, she hasn't seen the Brother eat since she arrived. Had we? Hmmm . . . The Lady said she got so wrapped up in planning Thanksgiving that, come to think on it, she hadn't seen him eat either—not for a week maybe. Taking care of himself now, we don't always see him feed himself, but the remnants of empty supplement cans are in the trash when he does. Nope, haven't seen any cans lately. He doesn't listen to the Lady, but we're not about to let him just wither and sleep his life away. Knowing he had an afternoon appointment at the cancer center on Monday, we drove there in the morning to let them know what's happening. The Lady asked if they'd please talk to him without letting him knowing we were there.

Yours,

Frog

♦ ♦ ♦ ♦ ♦ ♦ ♦ ♦

DECEMBER 6, 2010

Dear Family,

A large, glittery Christmas tree has been erected by the entrance of the cancer center. A bejeweled blitz, weighted down in garland, with a slight heavy hand used during the scattering of tinsel. In all its splendor, it's a wonderful welcome sight at the center. We love it! Sitting at the cancer center early this morning, we watch the patients start trickling in. Bundled up against the chill in the air, thin du-rags have now been replaced with heavier headgear. Ski caps in all colors dot the room. It's chemo week for the Sister. Looking around the room, there's such sickness in front of me. I notice the ones who are moving a little slower now and those who are a little thinner. It breaks my heart to witness these imperceptible transformations firsthand. I pray you never will. The Sister is not among these. She's gathered her strength and her walk is firm. I recognize the truth of the Lady's words; she doesn't walk alone. Looking pretty today in pink jeans and a black sweater, you could pass by her and not think she was sick. Today, the sisters giggle amongst themselves while waiting. Several eyes turn in our direction.

The Brother, devoting this part of his life to lying on the couch, will occasionally snap out of his recoil to join into the conversation. He's coming around, gradually. Really, he is. Rail-thin, a gaunt look has seized a grip on his face. It takes all his energy to rise, make his way to brush his teeth, returning to rest before gathering strength to rise again to shave. Ahhh, God love him. The surgeon's clinic has requested his presence on Thursday. The sisters, discussing this unexpected appointment, hope they'll speak to the Brother and tell him the importance of eating and gaining his strength to prepare for the future.

Three hours have passed quickly. The Lady and I move to a chair by the front door. Familiar faces and friends we haven't seen since back in radiation days pass by. It's a lovely day for a reunion.

Patients check in then come back to spend time with us before their appointments. Each face fills us with gladness. Even though time has kept rolling by, the fact that they now appear before us says they've all made it this far. Yes, today we see you! You're here! You're alive! Let's rejoice together, okay?

Another hour passes. Looking at the time, the Lady grabs her purse and satchel in haste as we race back to chemo. Wrapped up in seeing everyone, we'd forgotten to check on the Sister. She smiles when she sees us approach. My eyes follow the line that runs from the hanging empty pouch to the port in her chest.

"They just have to hook up my pump and we can GO!"

My gosh, I think to myself, *life is such a wonderful thing!*

Yours,

Frog

♦ ♦ ♦ ♦ ♦ ♦ ♦ ♦

DECEMBER 8, 2010

Dear Family,

It touched our hearts when the cancer center called to say they'd put the Brother and Sister on their Angel Tree list. Yesterday, the Sister was on the phone when I overheard her say, ". . . and candles and Christian books." She handed the phone to the Brother and he said, "sweats." He couldn't think of a single other thing. Believe me, he doesn't have much! He finally thought of mentioning nutritional supplements like Boost. It made me feel sad he couldn't think of anything more and the person on the other end of the line was having to work to come up with a list for him.

That's the thing about this family I'm staying with, they're always saying God is looking out for them. Sometimes, I'm convinced JPS and God are in cahoots together. I'm telling you, they just keep being a blessing to this family!

The Lady took me to see Santa. I told him about the cancer center's Angel Tree and *that*'s why I had to see him. If it wasn't too much trouble, on his way around the world could he please stop at the cancer center and drop off something especially nice for all those people?"

From this family to ours, have a wonderfully blessed Christmas!

Yours,

Frog

♦ ♦ ♦ ♦ ♦ ♦ ♦ ♦

DECEMBER 18, 2010

Dear Family,

I can't recall a greater lapse between letters than this one. I hope you haven't been worried about me. The Lady and I have been running all over the place preparing for Christmas. The sisters decorated their first tree together and it's done entirely in silver and dark purples—an interesting combination that screams success! The Lady's been baking cookies to send to her kids. Gifts are wrapped in silver-coordinating paper. She's adamant that everything must match and, half-kiddingly, instructed all household members to bring gifts to her and she'll wrap them for a nominal fee. This is a clear attempt to discourage anyone from sliding a green or red package under the tree that disrupts her color scheme. Did you get the gift I left on the front porch bench?

The Sister finished chemo again and got really discouraged when they handed her an appointment slip for her next treatment in January. Thinking she'd just finished her last treatment, she worries that her life will never get back to normal. She laid ill on the couch for days this time. Unopened mail piled beside her. Then one morning, with a smile on her face and wonderment in her voice, she called us over to her and told us to have a look at the Christmas card that arrived. If she'd been well, she would have trashed it days ago thinking it was the generic card she gets from her insurance agent. Instead, it was from the Cotopaxi Community Church Ladies' Bible Study group—complete strangers in another state who heard about her and wanted to send words of encouragement and a love gift. Our hearts fill to overflowing for this group of ladies. They made the Sister smile.

Now, on the flip side, a couple days later the Brother got his own card in the mail from a church. Careful in the opening of it so his check wouldn't fall between any cracks, he finds, instead, a printed form asking if he'd like to donate money to a charitable cause. We all laugh so hard saying it would've been the funniest thing if it had listed the special charity as the wonderful, sweet, angel of a person— (Sister's name). By the way, the Brother is doing so well now—happy every day and talking to us.

The Lady jumped out of bed last Saturday and hit her toe on a piece of furniture in the dark and almost broke it. Turning all black and purple, walking on it was unbearable. Unable to dress for church the next morning, she said she'd look like an idiot wearing flip flops with her dress slacks.

Remember how I told you this family keeps being provided for? Well, you remember way back when the refrigerator went out and a check was already in the mail to them from their Aunt Fran and Uncle Vernon who didn't even know the refrigerator was out? Sometimes you have to wait a little while because His timing is the perfect timing. Are you gonna panic or are you going to relax and let Him work His will? Last week, the Lady had to get her car serviced again. The morning before, she called to set up the appointment while we were sitting at the cancer center. That afternoon when we got home, in the mail was a card from her dealership for $15 off her next service. That card was already on its way before she had even thought to have the car serviced and it arrived just in time. A day later would've been too late. There's no such thing as too late when God is at work.

This morning, we met the Lady's son and girlfriend for breakfast in Ft. Worth at Old Neighborhood Grill by the hospital district. We'd never met Sarah before. Weeks ago, the Dad (after after speaking with his grandson) told the Lady to be prepared—this could be "the one." Sarah is just a tiny wisp of a thing and cute as can be. The four of us had a great time together with the girls hitting it off immediately. Walking outside to leave, Kyle and Sarah produce two beautiful boxes done in solid white with elaborate white ribbon and bows. I breathe a sigh of relief—it's a match with the tree!

Love,

Frog

♦ ♦ ♦ ♦ ♦ ♦ ♦ ♦

DECEMBER 25, 2010

Merry Christmas, My Dear Family!

This is a really special time for the siblings. On Thursday, the Lady and I went to the cancer center to get the Angel Tree gifts for the Brother and Sister. We walked out with a big stack of presents. We'd never met the woman who helped carry them to the car, but we stood in the parking lot talking to her for a while. She said every morning a group of employees gather for prayer for the staff and patients. The Lady got excited over that news because perhaps we can join them one morning. The woman also said, "I got to meet your dad when your parents were here." It feels like a blessing when people talk about the Dad; they recognize he's such a special man and it's not just our biased opinion.

Friday, a shipment of Ensure was delivered to the house for the Brother. It doesn't say who the angel was who sent it. It could have been any number of people—the cancer center or maybe even Santa himself!

Donna called last week from a store in New Jersey. She was having a hard time finding paper to match the tree since the Lady is such a stickler about it. Sending us three boxes of presents, all wrapped in silvers and purples, I'd say she was successful. The Sister's paper says *To Have, To Hold, To Love, To Cherish*. Wedding paper for Christmas? Yes! Why not? We love the wonderful zany feeling of it! Knowing the Lady, this could very well be the start of a new tradition.

Love,

Frog

♦ ♦ ♦ ♦ ♦ ♦ ♦ ♦

JANUARY 2, 2011

Dear Family,

It's officially a new year! I think it's safe to say, last year was a different year for all of us. During the past eight months of writing home, I've shared with you various people who have come into the lives of this family. Some people touched our lives just in passing, but their encouragement made a tremendous impact. Others are a constant, faithful presence. A complete list of each and every person who has given us encouragement could never be compiled. That would be impossible because there are so many, MANY special people.

Hello 2011! These people are loved, I'm loved, and you are loved.

Happy New Year!

Frog

♦ ♦ ♦ ♦ ♦ ♦ ♦ ♦

JANUARY 5, 2011

Dear Family,

Well, here we go. It's chemo week again. Monday, the Sister was hooked up to her pump. Never having recovered from the nausea from her last treatment, they drained a pouch of Ativan into her port before hooking up the portable pump. Liquid Ativan makes her loopy. We're not sure if it controls the nausea or if it just puts her in a state of *Eh, who cares?* She'll rise and sway in a stupor out to the car. The Lady, hooking their arms together, walks with her. Then the Sister will sleep the afternoon away. This had always been the drill in the past, until now.

On *this* Monday, we dropped her off at the house, drove to the post office, drove right back, and entered the house with the song *Girls Just Wanna Have Fun* by Cyndi Lauper playing. Well, actually blaring. What on earth? Since the Brother was also away, in privacy the Sister decided to try out the Wii *Just Dance* workout video he got her for Christmas.

"You gotta try it," she says to us, "just imitate the dance moves you see on TV and it'll score you."

The Lady strapped a hand-held remote to her hand and next thing we know, the rap song *U Can't Touch This* by MC Hammer was blaring. At first, struggling before getting the hang of it, the Sister says to her, "Oh! It says you're doing great on that one move." After hearing such encouragement, the Lady thought, *Oooooooh yeeeeaaaah! Look at me! MAN, I'm gooood!* When the song finished, it scored her as Great 7 percent of the song and Good 14 percent of the song and the other percent? Let's just say, having now seen her dance, it scores accurately.

Speaking like she'd just run a 5k with no break, all the while carrying a cinder block in her arms, she declines a second dance. Flopping down on the bed in exhaustion, while trying to catch her breath and steady her heart that threatened to pound right out of her chest and never return due to abuse, it wasn't pretty by any means. I'm quite sure she wouldn't appreciate me telling you exactly the extent of her out-of-shapeness, any more than telling you that the song was set on the Easy/Short version! What I'm trying to say is, the Sister held strong and woke up the next day with a radiant glow about her.

A week ago Tuesday, we went to the hospital with the Brother for his third biopsy. Afterward, the nurse came and led us back to where he was recovering. I was nervous about his appearance and told the Lady maybe she should say something because this was the worst he's looked after a biopsy. So she said to the nurse, "This is the *worst* he's looked after a biopsy!" Blood was pooled in the corner of his mouth. He was unconscious, yet tears were falling from the sides of his eyes. I didn't know that could happen while unconscious and was worried that this was a preview of the pain he'd be in once we got him home. No telling what we'd be in for! It surprised us both that, by the time they wheeled him out to the car, he was doing well.

He got the biopsy results yesterday. They remain unchanged— probable stage one carcinoma. The game plan? Come back in three weeks for a fourth biopsy and continue to biopsy to monitor his mouth. PET scan results are extremely accurate. If the PET scan says something is going on, you can pretty much rely on that. Either way, we feel very comfortable they aren't going to do a radical neck resection unless it's necessary.

Sitting for her five-hour treatment yesterday, the Sister was the last patient of the day at the cancer center on chemo side.

Day two is ending and the Sister is strong!

Yours,

Frog

◆ ◆ ◆ ◆ ◆ ◆ ◆ ◆

JANUARY 7, 2011

Dear Family,

A woman walks across the room to take a seat on chemo side. The Lady is immediately captivated by her. She bears an uncanny resemblance to a close friend the Lady lost touch with over 25 years ago. Living in Oklahoma, both were young moms in their early 20s. Remembering the fits of laughter they shared, the Lady smiles. Gosh! She hasn't thought of Lori in *years*! All of sudden, she misses her.

The woman takes a call on her cell phone. A second call will be from her 17-year-old son. (We later learn she has two very young children, as well.) Not meaning to intentionally eavesdrop, but unavoidable since she sits so near, the words are not what draw us in. It's her tone of voice. This voice represents a person with grace and a generous heart—very loving and kind. Catching part of the conversation ". . . *this weekend we'll go to the movies, okay? Just you and I . . .* " Her tone leaves little doubt this will be a special date between the two and she's excited about it.

It was just the most natural thing for the women to start talking to each other. She's fretting because chemo is so far behind schedule today. It's a school holiday and her young children are at a daycare. She promised she'd take them to the park to play. She *promised*! Yes, this woman's very much like the Lady. Her kids associate Mom as reliable and dependable. Keeping her word means everything. The two would continue to seek each other out for three consecutive days, both hunting the center down for the other. The Lady, one day, accidentally calls her "Lori" and they laugh. We like this woman and realize we'd never have gotten the chance to meet her if the Sister's schedule hadn't been delayed that week back in November. We would have missed out on something; we feel sure of this.

We want you to meet Kim, our new friend. She's vivacious, energetic, and gorgeous. Anyone who looks at her sees the undeniable picture of health and beauty and life itself! Kim has stage four cancer.

Already completing a round of chemo and radiation, she's now going through chemo treatments for a second time. She is classified as SO much more than warrior status. She is a fighter—a survivor!

Yours,

Frog

♦　♦　♦　♦　♦　♦　♦　♦

JANUARY 8, 2011

Dear Family,

This is the first letter I've written where the Lady said I would
have to wait to mail it. If I mailed it today, we might as well drive
right over to you, hold your hand, and lead you straight to the Sister—
blowing their cover. I guess I divulged too much information. My,
how quickly things can change in a day! Day Two—strong. Day
Three—not so good. We left early for the cancer center. The Sister
was suffering with sharp stomach pain and gut-wrenching vomiting.
Shaky, cold chills required her to leave the house wearing two layers
of clothing, a heavy coat, and a blanket wrapped around the whole
ensemble. The Sister is running a fever, so treatment is stopped and a
room is made ready for her on the 7th floor at JPS—Room 711. We're
glad it's room 711 for who knows *what* reason. Maybe the sound of
it—*oh thank heaven for 7-11.* Maybe it's because two blocks down
the street is the 7-11 the Lady raced to that one day to get snacks
for the Sister. The Lady's relieved with Dr. Choufani's decision. It's
not that she doesn't want to take care of the Sister, no, never that.
She feels inadequate. Accomplishing nothing by standing outside the
bathroom door, quietly knocking, asking if she needs help, a wash
cloth, or ice water. It's really an awful feeling when the gesture or
scenario is stuck on repeat. It wears you down.

Night descended, but with admission papers from the cancer
center in hand, we were going to be able to go straight to the 7th
floor. The Lady already had it planned to the Sister's advantage. The
parking garage was not an option since it was too far and too cold
outside. Also, the Sister is too ill. The small circle drive on the west
side of the building was perfect and closest to the bank of elevators
they would need. However, after going around the circle drive, only
one tiny spot was available—the #3 spot just before you complete the
circle. Stopping next to it, the Sister says she thinks the car will fit.
Our first attempt left us still hanging out in the driveway. Anxious, the

Lady got out of the car and tapped on the window of the man in spot #2, scaring him since he was minding his own business while fiddling with his phone.

"Sir, my sister's sick and being admitted on the 7th floor. I need to get her in through this door (pointing). Would you mind pulling out and going around the circle then parking behind me? (Pause while listening) Thank you! Thank you sooo much!"

I believe he handled the request well, considering the Lady might as well have cut to the chase and said, "I stink big time at parallel parking under nervous and tight situations. Pretty please, can I have *your* spot while you drive around the circle and have a go at it behind my car?" Well, that kindly gentleman pulled out of his spot and was giving it gas to go around the circle when he got even with the truck in the #1 spot. Suddenly, the truck's engine started up and drove away before the kindly man could stop his momentum and that's right, we ended up in the #1 spot. Divine intervention! No one could have predicted that happening, but we needed a spot and were given several.

The next morning, the Lady rose early to get ready to return to the hospital only to discover the kneecap on her right leg was useless. With no underlying reason at all, her knee felt like it'd been smashed with a baseball bat, although she doesn't personally know what that feels like. Unable to walk on it without immense pain, she nearly panicked. That's her driving leg and the Sister's in downtown Ft. Worth. She accidentally woke the Brother as she tried to maneuver through the dark house while using the wall for support. Getting up and making his way to her, she explained she'd be needing his cane. He helped her back to bed, retrieved the cane from his car, then placed it beside her. She laid down and silently started saying, "I am healthy! I am strong! I am well! God is good!" Over and over, she said this about 50 times. About half way through her mental chant, she had calmed down entirely, and her feather pillow started feeling especially inviting. Minutes later, sitting up and sliding the cane out of the way, she got up and felt no pain in her knee. None. I suggested we take the cane with us to the hospital just in case but she said we would NOT. That shows lack of faith. She needed her leg today and He gave her today.

I've been watching the Sister as I write this letter. It's 10:20 a.m. and she still sleeps. We've never seen her sleep this late. Even on the worst of days, she's an early riser. It seems she's hardly moved since we left her last night. Her blanket from home is still draped across her upper body. The portable spit-up bag is at her side. Her wig and du-rag sit perfectly on her head. I wish you could see her right this minute. She's an angel—a sleeping angel. Perhaps she was up all night. Neither one of us are willing to wake her to find out. So I say let her sleep because what we don't know is, later today they'll do chest and abdominal CT scans on her. Tomorrow, tomorrow they'll tell us her tumors are growing. The liver ones are probably causing her fever. The liver. Live-er. (A sob escapes aloud, time passes.)

A team of doctors tell us the upsetting news. Once they leave, facing away from us, the Sister turns on her side in a fetal position. The Lady grabs a tissue from the box. Going around to the other side of the bed, she presses it into the Sister's hand and says with conviction, "Oh no! We're not going to lose our faith. It's the Ativan making you weepy. We're going to stay strong!" Quickly excusing herself, she says we're going downstairs to McDonald's for lunch but, instead, the Lady changes her mind. We proceed down to the hospital lobby so she can be a hypocrite in private. Taking a seat among strangers, she cries openly. Making our way back to the bank of elevators, we hear, "Princess!" Turning to wave with a wobbly smile at Raymond in the distance, we keep walking.

"PRINCESS!" repeats Raymond.

Turning back around, she walks over to him and he gives her a hug and tells her in times like these, we've got to pray.

She is healthy. She is strong. She is well. God is good! She is healthy. She is strong. She is well. God is good! She is . . .

Yours,

Frog

♦ ♦ ♦ ♦ ♦ ♦ ♦ ♦

JANUARY 14, 2011

Dear Family,

Certainly news of the tumors growing has caused a temporary set back in emotional well-being among the sisters. The morning after returning home from the hospital, they meet in the kitchen. The Sister confides she's tired of washing her wig all the time. Will her life ever go back to the way it was before she got sick? Another thing she's been thinking about is how sad it is that other people buy books to read for enjoyment and she's buying books trying to find out how to live longer. She starts to cry.

The Lady thinks about this, the Sister's sorrow, and thinks about dying. It's not so much the Sister doesn't want to *ever* die—it's just she's not ready to right now. Long ago, she told the Lady she still has so much more she wants to do in life. I wonder if there's ever a point you reach where you confidently announce that right now, today, I'd like to die. Maybe after endless days of enduring intense pain, such thoughts might be induced. The Lady, personally, has no fear of dying at any given moment. She believes that you live forever starting on the very day you accept salvation. Sometimes we have to be reminded that forever doesn't start on the day you die when you're a Christian. Preferably, death won't be any time soon for the Lady so she can continue helping the siblings over this phase in their lives. But, the Sister? No, she doesn't want to die—not today—not for a while. It scares her. Do you know how I know that? The longest letter I wrote home, the part where the sisters don't break eye contact? The staring, staring, eternity part? Remember the unspoken words you hear with your eyes? It was her eyes; they told us. Placing her arm around the Sister, the Lady reminds her, "I am healthy. I am strong. I am well. God is good. Say it and keep *on* saying it!" The Sister agrees, this is 2011 so she'll only think good things for all of us this year.

Wednesday, the sisters and I met with Dr. Choufani to find out where we go from here. The Sister finished six rounds of Cisplatin (that five-hour serious drug). He tells us the treatment worked exceptionally well, far better than expected. The Sister looks good and her weight is still holding. Because the tumors are now growing, this tells him her body is no longer responding to that treatment. He wants to speak with the hospital doctor who does chemo treatments directly to the liver and see if he'll accept her. It's a two-day hospital stay and, usually, if cancer is anywhere else in the body, they don't feel the treatment would be beneficial. However, since her cancer is primarily in the liver now, he'll see if they'll consider it.

The Lady asks what if they won't do the procedure? Then what? (The Sister is eating healthy! She exercises when she can. She bought a juicer to start juicing. She's reading all these books and praying—so much praying! So listen, listen to me . . . We're following all the rules, ALL of them. Give us something. Whatever you're about to say, remember we're following the rules. That's gotta count for *something*, right?)

Here's the part that I, along with the sisters, notice. When Dr. Choufani turns to serious matters that drag in emotional reactions, he'll quietly and repeatedly clear his throat.

Well . . . (clear throat) *we will give her a couple weeks break and then start chemo trying some* (clear throat) *different drugs. We're going to fight this together, (Sister's name), you and me* (clear throat) *to the end.*

The Lady was staring intently at his face as he spoke and, as if to conclude the visit with . . . *to the end* still hovering around in the atmosphere, a huge tear over-spilled from the middle of her left eye, free-falling off her cheek due to the weight of it, onto her coat. All three of us were lost in our own thoughts, which happened to be the exact same thought: You've got to LOVE this doctor. You just gotta!

Yours,

Frog

◆   ◆   ◆   ◆   ◆   ◆   ◆   ◆

JANUARY 19, 2011

Dear Family,

The first time she said it, we completely ignored the statement as simply preposterous. It was about as likely, in our estimation, as her declaring she'd awakened that morning to discover her hair had grown out over night resembling a perfectly coiffured beehive, deep red in color. *See?* The following day she repeated herself as we lounged in the living room. "I've been thinking about stopping treatment." We look her way, tongue-tied. "I honestly am!" A speech spills forth that mimics the same conviction and force an attorney would use, designed to change the minds of jurors, swaying them into his or her corner. She's looking for an ally in the room. We're certainly at a loss for words and make polite comments to show interest without committing ourselves to joining the team—just yet.

The chemo is killing her, she says. As long as it's in her system she won't ever feel well. Good days have become a thing of the past. She thinks she has nerve damage, numbness in her limbs, and the occasional ringing in her ears is now a constant. Several weeks ago, the ringing in her ears was an on-again off-again thing. We visited JPS second floor for a hearing test which, at that time, indicated the Sister's hearing was fine. Closed in a sound booth with her back positioned to us, the Sister pressed a button every time she heard a noise through her headset. At the end of the test, the technician handed her own headset to the Lady to put on. She spoke into the sound booth, "Whatsoever you ask in My name it shall be done for you."

The Sister's convinced if the chemo were expelled from her body, she'd be a normal functioning human again. Her old self would return. She's been reading about alternative cancer treatments with a more natural approach such as juicing (which she recently started), green smoothies, asparagus, and raw honey. Next, she shares miraculous success stories from survivors. Some were stage four, just like her, who are perfectly healthy now after using these other methods. Still no cancer after 10, 12, 14 or whatever years later.

The Lady's friend, Mary, in Florida, was the first person to share with her the importance of a raw diet. Green smoothies! Green smoothies! If anyone would know, it'd be Mary. The two women met over a year ago in Guatemala at an orphanage. Both were going through difficult trials in their lives and wanted to give back to others rather than concentrate on the difficulties of their own lives. (The Lady interrupted, wanting me to tell you if ever you start feeling sorry for yourself, turn your focus on what you can do for others. Remember, life's not all about *me*.) Anyway, the Lady thought Mary was simply a marvelous person! Mary thought the same about her and, ever since then, they're like sisters.

Mary, God bless her, has a medical history that'd scare the most fearless person. In 2003, she had non-Hodgkins lymphoma with a tumor the size of your fist that paralyzed a vocal cord. Her voice is raspy, but in a totally good, sultry-sounding way, which the Lady wishes hers could resemble although not as the result of a tumor. Mary underwent chemo and radiation at that time. In 2008, she had a benign tumor the size of a golf ball on the left side of her brain (the part that controls speech) removed. Also, that year, she had an implant put in her neck to help her vocal cord. Because of all she's gone through, it led her to find a better way to take care of her body and she became interested in the raw food diet.

In private, the Lady says she'd love to believe in alternative treatments. Maybe when she reads the books herself, as she plans to soon, she'll have more faith that organic coffee enemas can reject and eliminate tumors completely. Certainly, the Sister has every right to make her own choices as to what's best for her. We'd like to do everything in our power to assist in alternative treatments as long as it's also part of her current doctor-controlled treatment. Oh, who are we to say, though? It's not our place. What do we know? Not much, really, any more.

The Lady has half a mind to tattle again to the chemo office. Perhaps they can talk with the Sister and help her with her decision. The only reservation we have about following through with that is the stark fear that the doctor or nurse will accidentally (or not) be forced to explain if treatment stops, you can expect X amount of time left. We all agreed early on that we wanted none of that. No time frames revealed. Sure, we hear people say, *I was given six months to live, and that was 18 months ago . . .* However, we don't believe it's healthy to be told a time frame because, even if you become indignant and declare, "Pffff!!!! I don't believe that for one minute!" that seed of time is still planted in your subconscience. It has to screw with you some. A sure faith-buster.

The Sister won't do anything without thinking it over very seriously from all angles. Of this, we're sure. In the meantime, I guess we'll just assist however we can, starting now, by loading up the coffee pot with some of that organic stuff.

Yours,

Frog

♦　♦　♦　♦　♦　♦　♦　♦

JANUARY 24, 2011

Dear Family,

Why *sure* by the looks of her in the Thanksgiving picture, you'd believe Donna was as healthy as a horse. That all changed one morning when the Lady opened an e-mail from her titled: *A New Medical Issue to Watch For.*

The way she told it, she was eating one night when a piece of food ended up under her tongue. While reaching to pull the food out, she felt two large lumps. After closely examining them in the mirror, then insisting other members of the household open their mouths for comparison, she determined two large horns were growing under her tongue which, characteristic to this family, totally freaked her out!

If this solely involved Donna, I'd have a tendency to continue with the story as is. However, I'm bringing the Lady's version into it now and, due to the delicate nature of this abomination, she told me it'd probably be best if I didn't repeat any of it. Since you're my family and I can attest to the fact you're not a bunch of blabbermouths, I feel comfortable relaying this in confidence. You can certainly see their hesitation with news of this magnitude leaking. With both of them being single women, what hope could they possibly have finding a future mate with this "condition" hanging over their heads?

Several years ago, the Lady's mouth was hurting badly under her tongue. She, too, investigated it in the mirror and was alarmed at what she saw. (Suggestion: Don't ever look in a 10x magnifier unless applying makeup.) It looked like she had two new teeth wanting to punch through at the age of 40-something. It hurt like bothersome wisdom teeth. She was convinced if she showed Dr. Glover, she'd be asked to accompany him to the next annual American Dental Association conference (where she'd be the star specimen) so they could all view this medical oddity. Then the following year, clearly without her permission, her open mouth would be plastered in the *Guinness World Records* book where kids who weren't raised better would snicker at her as they nudged their friends and said, "Check out the lady on page 78!" Besides all that, is there a clause on her dental insurance plan that clearly states Dental Oddities are not covered?

The Lady ended up asking Dr. Glover, "What *are* those *things*?" (She'd never call them horns!) They were calcification that form in the mouth, usually stress-related. Donna, not knowing at the time the Lady had issues in the same department, encouraged her to look up the medical term online. I still hold firm with the Lady's belief, as long as you don't know about a disease it can't *possibly* happen to you! So, as a precaution, I'd discourage you from doing further Internet research on this.

The next morning, we received a text from Donna, drained after only getting two hours of sleep from worrying about the horns. She'd neglected to research exactly how large they can grow. We all ended up laughing about it, especially after Donna found out she wasn't the only one suffering. The Dad, reluctantly admitting he was also afflicted, agrees this can be part of a Frog letter provided no photos of him prior to 1990 are attached. The Lady wisely counsels Donna that she should be fine as long as she avoids, at all costs, touching her tongue to her nose in public. Donna, ever one to remain positive, ends the discussion with the following text:

Face it. It could be worse. They could be growing on my forehead!

Yours,

Frog

♦　♦　♦　♦　♦　♦　♦　♦

JANUARY 26, 2011

Dear Family,

I hope you take notice of shortcuts as the Lady and I discovered well over six months ago. Sometimes they lead down roads you're meant to travel, roads that bear gifts for the person who pays attention. That's what happened to the Lady when she decided to cut through an upscale neighborhood to get to CVS Pharmacy. What initially seemed like a time-saver, turned out to be more. There's one house that makes a statement to us and all others who follow this same path. These homeowners have the boldness to not care what the world thinks, but what God thinks. This family has their priorities in order. They can only hope their message lifts spirits, brings comfort, and serves as a reminder to others not to forget to check their priorities. The home is on a lovely street made even lovelier when you take a moment to gaze upon the black wrought iron gate that crosses their drive. Eyes of strangers who diligently search for the gate each time, read the following: *SEEKING GOD'S OWN HEART.* I wonder how many people it must influence by speaking directly to hearts?

This particular gate has become a landmark for the Lady and I. The Lady never misses a chance to slow the car to a lazy roll to read it once again. It's still there. Nothing's changed. The Lady sighs in relief. Her family is in God's heart and He in theirs. It wasn't until Christmas arrived that she shared the story of this gate with another, prompted by receiving a Christmas present, a simple bangle bracelet with a loopy design in the middle. If you look closely, it spells GOD in the shape of a heart—God's heart! My word, she gets excited and rushes to LifeWay and buys the Brother and Sister a God's heart lapel pin to wear daily as a reminder to keep God close to their hearts. She vows, in the future, to continue passing out as many of these pins as she can.

She believes for some reason we're supposed to meet the people who own this gate. She wants to tell them that they're part of our journey and they don't even know it. It weighs on her mind that perhaps no one takes the time to tell them their gate is special to others. The holidays come and go and no time seems appropriate. Someday, she promises, she'll do it. Someday she'll march right up to that front door and ring the bell. Yet, more time passes. Her heart continues telling her to do this but, quite frankly, she's nervous about the whole idea. It sounds so much easier to fulfill while lying around in bed at night thinking about it. Several times, we get in the car to complete the task, slow to a crawl in front of the house, and then fear seizes her and we race off like maniacs.

Last week, a package arrived in the mail from Renee'. Opening it, gladness fills the Lady's heart. Totally unaware of this story and acting on the belief this is something the Lady needs, she was compelled to send a bracelet made up of a solid circle of God's Hearts. As if any more confirmation were really needed, on Sunday, the pastor closed the service by saying he wanted to give everyone an opportunity to become a part of God's heart. The Lady's eyes got huge, nudging her sisters, she mouths, "God's heart! He just *said* it!"

Such a story, a gate that impacts lives, unprecludable signs—all are heaven-sent. Two families, unknown to each other, sharing the love of the same gate and the same heart.

Yours,

Frog

♦　♦　♦　♦　♦　♦　♦　♦

Dear Family,

Quite a bit has happened this past week, but I'll have to write about it later. I was holed up in the Lady's borrowed room for almost four days while she suffered a sinus headache. (Boring!) I don't have much time to write because we have running around to do. Don't worry about her, though, I knew she was definitely on the mend when she woke up this morning and said, "Is it just *me* or do my legs look skinnier."

I do have to quickly tell you one thing that happened. A couple months ago, we were having coffee with Ken and Lu Ella at I-HOP when Lu Ella said she found some pink glasses at a garage sale and thought of the Lady. She'd heard the story of the pair that got run over in the CVS parking lot. Framed in rhinestones with a couple missing, she'd give them to her if she wanted them. Pink rhinestones, you say? The Lady wanted them!

Last weekend, Donna arrived from New Jersey to celebrate her birthday with us. On Saturday, all of us, except the Brother, headed over to visit Ken and Lu Ella at their house. Their son, Steve, was there so it was kind of a reunion. Donna and the Sister hadn't seen them since the 70s. When it came time to leave, the Lady said, "Hey, where are those glasses?" Lu Ella went around the corner and came back placing an eyeglass case in her hand. The Lady immediately said, "Ohhh! This case feels really nice!"

Days later, she pulled the glasses out to investigate them closely. The first time she opened the case, she noticed there was a perfectly scrolled piece of paper off to one side. Assuming it was to help prevent the glasses from jostling around, for some reason she decided to unscroll it. It revealed a typed message: READ ROMANS 8:23. Why Lu Ella! It's just like her to send a secret message. She thumbs through her Bible and reads verses 23 through 27 then shares the verses with the Sister since they speak of hope.

Lady (texting Lu Ella): btw did u leave me a little typed message in the eyeglass case? Loved that.

Lu Ella: What did it say??

Lady: It read: READ ROMANS 8:23 u didnt do that?

Lu Ella: No. I never unfolded the paper. You will laugh at me, but I thought the lady who owned the glasses put that in there to replace a missing piece. HA!

I found the whole I'm-tucking-a-secret-message-into-my-old-eyeglass-case-before-I-give-them-away concept intriguing. Who *is* this woman and what's the story behind her actions? Regardless of the means, another message was delivered with success.

Yours,

Frog

♦ ♦ ♦ ♦ ♦ ♦ ♦ ♦

FEBRUARY 11, 2011

Dear Family,

We spent part of Monday morning at an attorney's office to see about having a will drawn up for the Sister. That wasn't easy; I could tell. However, the Sister said she felt much better taking care of that. Later that day, the Sister, Lady, and I went to JPS Hospital to meet with a surgeon who reviewed the Sister's case to see if she qualifies for chemo treatment directly to the liver. Dr. Choufani told us there was a chance this doctor wouldn't accept her since she has cancer in more places than her liver, so we were nervous about what he was going to tell us. He showed us a scan of five tumors on her liver and said he believes this treatment (chemoembolization) will benefit her.

Next week, she'll spend the night at the hospital. They're going to go through an artery in her leg, up to her liver, and follow the vein that leads to each tumor. They'll inject three chemo drugs into each tumor then close the artery off. Blood flowing to tumors feeds them so it's necessary to stop the blood supply. Once the tumor starts to die, it releases toxins into the system and can make a person very sick. The doctor showed us before and after shots from other patients and it's amazing to see really large tumors almost gone within a matter of months. One patient had so many tumors. *See this patient?* (We looked hard at the screen.) *This person had about three months to live before treatment and that was over a year ago.* I couldn't help but wonder who that person was and hoped he or she was now leading a happy life. Maybe someday another person will be looking at the Sister's liver as the surgeon tells them how well she did. She could be a success story. She could make it! After she has this treatment, she'll see this surgeon every three months from now on for monitoring.

The Sister's so brave and so strong to go through everything she's gone through. I'm proud of her because sometimes I lie in bed at night and scare myself with worry. What if I had to go through what she has? Someday, I want you to meet her so you can see how sweet she is.

You'd love her. For the past two weeks, she keeps telling the Lady and I she wants all of us to go to heaven—ALL of us—and all their kids and family. Then she says she wants everyone in the world to go and prays for every person on earth! This shocked the Lady and made her feel strange that she never thought to pray for the whole entire world herself. Come to think about it, it's mostly all geared to people she knows and it never dawned on her to broaden her request universally. This just shows how much the sisters learn from each other.

Tuesday, we were back on the second floor of JPS Hospital to see about the results from the Brother's fourth biopsy. They've decided to redo the PET scan now. The biopsies aren't turning up anything so they want to make sure the PET scan was accurate. They also told him they wouldn't be able to fix his jaw. He had hopes there was something they could do to make his jaw work so he could eat. We were half-expecting him to kick something on our way out, but he seemed to take the news in stride and said he's going to start exercising it and *make* it work. He came home later in the day with a bag of McDonald's french fries and was trying to gnaw on the limp ones. He confessed to trying to eat a spoonful of Manwich the night before but couldn't control it, which can be very dangerous. Half his mouth has no feeling, and his jaw only opens the width of a toothbrush. Do you know what it's like when you go to the dentist and they numb your mouth? Once, the Lady almost killed herself because she didn't want to wait to eat after going to the dentist. With her mouth numb, she tried to eat a bowl of skinny noodles and choked so hard she thought, *This is IT. This is my demise. This is how it's going to go down, with my obituary reading I died from a noodle!*

The Lady and I were going to vacuum her car, but before we knew what hit us we found ourselves pulling into a place that makes breakfast croissants that are to die for. They make them all day long with just the right amount of too much grease! I would highly recommend you try one. We got you the new winter antenna topper because we noticed the one on your car is faded. When we showed it to the Sister, she started laughing and pointed out that it looks like he's wearing a du-rag just like her! We loved it and hope you do too.

Yours,

Frog

♦   ♦   ♦   ♦   ♦   ♦   ♦   ♦

Dear Family,

God help us! The Lady's conscience is shredded over something she did and she doesn't know how to find peace over this. Remember when they hospitalized the Sister last month because she got so sick during chemo treatment? On the day we were to bring the Sister home, there was a stack of discharge paperwork lying on the hospital window sill. The Lady stuffed everything into the overnight bag. That night, she pulled the papers out and saw there were complete reports of CT scans the Sister has had since April when she was first hospitalized. We read over the reports, and it's a progression of her tumors. In April, the radiologist listed the location and size of her tumors. Then she had scans in May, July, November, and January. At first, it was interesting because the radiologist noted in the earlier scans new tumors and the enlarging of old tumors. Then there was the remarkable November scan where the tumors were shrinking or gone. We got to January's report that showed the tumors are now growing. Anyway, what I'm getting at is, the Lady hid the report from the Sister with full intention of letting her read it if she were ever to ask, which she hasn't. The action of burying the report in her closet was because the Lady knew the Sister would scour it with the same critical eye she did to try and determine how fast each tumor grew in a month and a half. That was the only reason; the Lady didn't want her doing that.

You may wonder what the problem is. It started with the first follow-up visit with Dr. Choufani when the Sister told him her liver tumors were growing. The Lady almost said something at that time but held her tongue. A few weeks later, at a follow-up visit with the radiation doctor, the Sister told the nurse her liver tumors are growing. At home, she'd discussed on more than one occasion *that* fact, but we realize she totally doesn't know the original tumor is also growing. The Lady followed the nurse out of the examination room, touched her arm to get her attention, then explained the Sister doesn't know her other tumor is growing. Adding, at this point, she doesn't know how to tell her. The nurse says she understands and sometimes, for whatever reason, some don't tell.

We were all in the hospital room the morning the head doctor came in with about six resident doctors in tow. He looked at the Sister, then at the Lady, and said, "You're sisters! No sense trying to lie about it! (laughter) We compared your CT scan from yesterday to the one in November and your tumors are growing. The liver tumors, I believe, are causing your fevers." Maybe it was in that instant the Sister heard nothing but *liver tumors* resounding in her head and it was all her mind registered from that point on. I can only guess.

Thursday, the sisters sat quietly throughout the day, each reading their own copy of the book, *Flight to Heaven* by Capt. Dale Black. It's a book Donna sent that talks about physical healing and a man's account of visiting heaven. It was a really nice day until the Lady went to take off her makeup and started thinking about how the Sister looked sitting on the couch, all unsuspecting and innocent. The Lady felt as if this were just the most saddest thing ever—secrets that go beyond fingers pressed to lips to silence news of high fevers.

The Lady will think about her actions at night while lying in bed, and she'll punch the mattress with her fist in frustration that maybe she's made a mistake and the Sister deserves to know. What if she tells her and it makes her lose hope and causes more damage than if she never even knew? It could happen. Your mind can mess with your health. A perfect example was yesterday. The Sister got up and worked out for a while on her treadmill. Later, we all walked into the cancer center, another *good* day until we asked for the lab results from her last visit and this visit. The last visit was odd because they said we couldn't have the results as they were sent over to the main hospital lab for them to rerun. "Why's that?" we asked at the time. It was because a reading was "off" and they needed to double check it.

So, of course, this week we wanted to get our hands on those results to see for ourselves. The Sister was sitting in a room on the exam table, as the Lady looked over the white blood count readings, informing us her count was excellent during chemo week. Normal range for white blood count is considered 4.3-10.8. The three days she was in the hospital show readings of 9.68, 8.15, and 6.36. Then it shows her last reading, the one we couldn't see at the time dipped way down to 2.98. At this point the Sister, who was previously fine, announced she didn't feel so well all of a sudden. "My white count must be off today too; that's the reason they sent it over to the hospital again!" She admits her mind is playing with her and maybe she should lie down. What would the people in the waiting room *think*? The ones who saw her arrive earlier but now see her leave in a wheelchair with a white blanket tucked around her, as the Lady runs to move the car as close to the entrance as possible to pick her up? We laughed like we'd never stop over that scenario, but there's truth to the saying: What you don't know can't hurt you.

The Lady confides to the Brother and Donna, "I mean, what good could come of it, right?" All the while, trying to find the one person who'll tell her it's okay and she'll actually believe them. Then there'll be no more punching the mattress at night and no more restlessness of her spirit.

Yours,

Frog

P.S. The cancer center is kicking off Relay For Life for the next couple months. The proceeds go to support the American Cancer Society and JPS cancer patients. Right now, they're selling long-sleeved shirts with their logo on it. It feels soft and comfy so the Lady bought one last month. Later that same day, when the Lady, Sister, and I were shown to a room, a CT technologist knocked on the door and said someone in the building heard we had bought a shirt so they bought a second one so both the Lady and the Sister each had one. She wouldn't tell us who was responsible for the kind gesture but we decided yesterday we want you to have a shirt, too.

♦ ♦ ♦ ♦ ♦ ♦ ♦ ♦

FEBRUARY 16, 2011

Dear Family,

    This should be what I consider another landmark letter, where I go into how many days the Lady and I have been gone, but it's not. In fact, I'm hardly even going to talk about this family because I'm supposed to tell you another story. I've thought of little else for the past couple days. You know how I *really* know I should tell you? Because earlier I was going to write to you about this, but instead I took a long nap, hardly able to rouse myself. I woke realizing the devil didn't want me telling people about this. In fact, he'd like nothing better than for the Lady and I to keep our mouths shut. Well, too bad!

    A couple weeks ago, Renee' sent the Lady a book called *Two Weak Women and Amazing Grace* by Bonnie Hanson. It's a wonderful account of two women (Alline and Bonnie) in their 50s who spent most of their lives abroad in the mission field until God sent them off in another direction. Two women, with barely two nickles to rub together, instructed by God to buy 55 acres in the northeast Georgia mountains and build a Christian retreat called Fellowship Valley—a place where many would come to salvation—a place that brings renewal to the souls of others. This was an amazing journey full of obstacles and faithful servants who saw their needs being met in His perfect timing.

    What makes this journey even more intriguing and personal is, over 30 years later, their friend Tina (whom the women have known since junior high) had a calling to be part of keeping this vision alive. She turned her back on the life she'd made for herself and was obedient to what God wanted this phase of her life to be. The Lady sent her an e-mail, and I want to share with you the return e-mail:

    Hey (Lady's first name),

    I'm so glad you got to read the book. It has been such an inspiration to so many people over the years, including myself, for sure! When things settle for you and the Sister, I invite both of you to come here and just "chill" in His presence! As a matter of fact, bring the whole family!

Below, is an excerpt of a letter I wrote to the surrounding communities, inviting them to be a part of what God is doing here. It kind of sums up my current involvement. I currently carry the title of "Operations Manager," which is a glorified title for "Volunteer Handymam for the Lord!" The Lord called me back here in April of 2010 and I've been "walking on water" with Him ever since. He meets all my needs and even blesses me with a couple of wants in the process. I am happier than I've ever been and I know I am right where He wants me to be in this journey.

What began over 32 years ago as a huge step of faith for Bonnie and Alline, continues today through the ministry of Fellowship Valley. God mightily used these "two weak women" to disciple a generation of believers of the Body of Christ through this ministry. Although Bonnie has gone Home to be with her Lord, and Alline has retired from the day-to-day involvement of the ministry, God is proving He is far from done with this awesome place, on the contrary!

From August of 2005 through January of 2007, Fellowship Valley was my "home" while I was dealing with, as well as recuperating from, some medical and financial issues. Bonnie and Alline were my Spiritual Mothers who took me in, cared for me, and nursed me back to "Faith." As the Lord lead me on from here to take care of my own family, I knew I would never forget the true Christian love that I experienced here during my time of need. Unbeknownst to me, God was not through with my connection here. In April of last year, the Lord called me back to Fellowship Valley to carry on the walk of faith that this place is known for, but not this time as someone who needed to be taken care of, but in the role of "caretaker!" I can promise you, there has never been a dull moment! Even while the Board is currently pursuing the task of qualifying more faith-filled believers to add to the leadership team here, (those who will stay the course and continue the "Vision" the Lord gave these women so many years ago) I have been blessed with the opportunity to serve Him by continuing the legacy as another "weak woman" willing to hear the Voice of the One who directs my steps, be obedient to that Voice, and do it all for His Glory, through the ministry of Fellowship Valley.

In the midst of Bonnie's passing and Alline's retirement, Fellowship Valley has gone through a dry season over the past couple *of years, allowing the Lord to position it for a renewed anointing. Because of the 32-year history of this beautiful place, we are not praying to "start from scratch," but to "start refreshed"—to stand in faith for God's Refreshing and Provision to permeate this 60 acres, with not only a continuation of His Vision, but to allow Him to expand that Vision in a new and exciting way.*

Well! I wanted to take off for Clarkesville, Georgia, after reading this, but our schedule wouldn't allow it. I told the Lady we need to see how we can still be involved and to please give me some of her money to send as support. I know this family doesn't have a lot of money to throw around, but the Lady tithes faithfully and because she's faithful, God always, always meets their needs. *Yes*, she said, *we can send something.* The more I thought about it, I decided there might be others out there who are going to feel led to send support too. How do you know if you're led? Because it stays on your heart and won't go away until you act. It's another obedience thing. I told the Lady if someone sends five dollars then tells others, and the others send something, this could be the greatest blessing! Pray about it, and if you decide to jump aboard, send a note telling Tina who you are and that you heard about Fellowship Valley from the Frog.

There is a second reason I knew I was supposed to tell you this story. Last night, I was writing to you like a mad maniac, words spilling forth almost faster than I could type, when the computer ripped all my words off the page and made them disappear. This has never happened before while writing to you. Disgusted, I ran and told the Lady to have a look, my letter was GONE! She immediately sent an e-mail to Tina telling her what happened and Tina replied:

You must be really tickin' him off! So, here we go...Satan, in the Name of Jesus, we cancel your assignment against the Frog and the purpose God has for him and we send you packing! Get lost!

Okay, brother, type away!

Yours,

Frog

P.S. I'm sending you the Lady's copy of *Two Weak Women and Amazing Grace.*

♦ ♦ ♦ ♦ ♦ ♦ ♦ ♦

FEBRUARY 18, 2011

Dear Family,

It was horrible. I never want to relive it. Our nerves were already jarred as we sat in the hospital's radiology waiting room while the Sister underwent chemoembolization to her liver. At 11:30 a.m., sirens screeched through the waiting area. Overhead strobe lighting flashed in brilliant bursts. Closing her book and removing her reading glasses, tears well in the Lady's eyes. Is this a huge God sign or what? What's going on? Was the Sister in trouble? PRAY!, she texts Donna. We were told early this morning the details of the procedure and learned that after chemo is injected into each tumor, they back out of the vein and release tiny beads into the bloodstream. These beads continue their journey with the flow of blood until they reach the tumor, creating a dam, sealing it off. Is that what did it? Did they fail to dam up, causing the Sister to go into cardiac arrest or something as we sit here? The sirens and lighting are unnerving. Scared beyond measure, we walk into the hallway and pull a staff member aside for reassurance. We're told that it's only the safety system being checked.

Hours later, we're led to the recovery room. The nurse says the procedure went extremely well, but the Sister's not being "a good patient." To us, she doesn't look well. We don't like this and want it to be yesterday once again. Take it all back. Redo our thinking. Delay what lays ahead to when we were unsuspecting and clueless of today. We're instructed to make sure she remains calm and doesn't move her right leg—the leg with the artery used for the procedure. The leg is strapped down. Even comatose, the Sister is not happy about it. It would be best if she could sleep through this. The nurse says not to encourage any talking. *Sleep, sleep, sleep,* we chant in our head. As if on cue, the nurse leaves and the Sister goes into a groggy fit. The Lady rushes to hold her down and whispers words of comfort— calling upon God. *Be with her!*

Every five minutes or so, the scenario is repeated again, and

The Frog Letters

again, and again. The Sister incoherently calls out the Lady's name, over and over, much as a child calls for his or her mother. *Mumbling. Mumbling. (Lady's name), it hurts!* Time passes. *(Lady's name), I'm sick.* Hearts start racing. "Shhhh! Sweetheart, you're doing so well!" *(God? I know you're here. Make it stop. Just please make this stop!)* She pauses without moving a muscle to evaluate the situation. *(Did it stop? No? Not yet? Well, it WILL! I have faith it will.)* It crushes our hearts as we keep racing to her side to still her leg. Words of comfort, prayers rush from lips, and fingers are crossed. All the wishbone wishes from years past are now taken back and thrown on this one moment.

The admitting physician is called to assess her and he immediately comes to her room. He says that the hospital is filled to capacity; they're stacking. *Stacking?* He explains this means patients are being lined in the hallways in beds. The Lady, pleading, asks him to please not let this happen to the Sister. *Can't we just stay here?* Unfortunately, this area closes at five. He leaves and we can hear him making phone calls from a nurse's station. A curtained off area is found on the third floor in the outpatient observation area. Shortly after, they transport the Sister there while we follow.

Once she's settled in, still unconscious, we escape downstairs to place quick phones calls and texts before the battery runs out on the phone. Rebecca, who works at the hospital, walks past and the women hug, happy to see each other. Like Raymond, we always manage to run into Rebecca. She's an inspiration and shares a story about her being obedient to God's will. We tell her we love her as we get up to leave. Thank God for the people He puts in our path.

We have to force ourselves to go back to the third floor. I know that sounds awful, but it feels so much safer sitting in the hallway chair outside McDonald's. Tubes have been removed from the Sister in our absence. She's quiet, unconscious really, until she starts mumbling the Lady's name over and over. Grabbing a portable spit-up bag, we rush to pull her unresponsive body into an upright position, holding the bag under her chin as she gets sick. Moments later, her head falls forward and she's out. We start to lay her back down when nearly the identical scene plays out again. We're ready; we've done this before. Shaky fingers adjust her wig while we have the chance, an important promise kept. A loud cry of pain fills the room. She's out.

Nine and a half hours ago, we were waiting for the Sister's name to be called for this procedure. Now, exhausted, we leave the building. We leave the Sister behind. She's not even aware we were there or that we are now gone. As we walk to the parking garage, neither of us is able to look at the other. Plagued by the same kind of guilt you might experience when you accidentally step on the paw of a beloved pet then hurriedly say, "I'm sorry! I'm sorry! I'm sorry!" Somehow, it never makes either feel any better.

Yours,

Frog

♦ ♦ ♦ ♦ ♦ ♦ ♦ ♦

FEBRUARY 22, 2011

Dear Family,

We set the alarm so we could race back to the hospital early Thursday morning, nervous about which nurse would be assigned to the Sister.

The day before, we sat squished in a chair in a tiny area designed to hold one bed and just enough walking room on either side. Our chair blocked off access to one side completely. The Lady sat with a blank stare directed at the curtain, lost in thought over what to do, all the while twirling her hair between her fingers—a nervous habit from childhood. I eavesdropped on the dialog from the TV of a nearby patient. It's a reality court show with a female judge. Someone was suing over a broken lease, and the other party was countersuing because of cockroaches. I was rooting for the cockroach people. Anyway, on that day, the nurse assigned to the Sister was mean to her—mean to an unconscious person! Can you even begin to grasp that concept? Since the Sister was totally defenseless, we couldn't do anything but sit there for hours and stand guard. Doing anything else, but guard her, was unthinkable. The whole thing was terribly upsetting. The Lady doesn't like confrontation but, due to exhaustion, she realizes she's not going to make it another hour and a half until shift change. Approaching the nurse's desk, she explains we must leave and then she bends close to the nurse and quietly says, "Please be nice to (Sister's name) while I'm gone." The nurse immediately ushered us out in the hall to confirm, *Why, of COURSE I will!* Unconvinced, but with no malice in her tone, the Lady tells her she wasn't at all happy over what took place earlier. Getting back to the house, I told the Lady to go on to bed while I sat and typed a two-page letter to the hospital administration letting them know what happened. The reason I tell you this story is because we never realized, before this happened, just how important it is to watch over loved ones when they're helpless and under the care of someone you don't know.

DianaRae

Thursday, when we arrived at the hospital, we were relieved the Sister had been assigned to Jennifer, a warm, caring nurse. It would be another four hours before the Sister would be discharged. She slipped in and out of consciousness during this time, never entirely "there."

Our drive home is slow; each bump or curve in the road awakens her to elicite cries of pain. Assisting her into the house, the Brother looks, then shakes his head slowly back and forth in sorrow, at her condition. "Morphine," she chokes out as we get her settled in her spot on the couch. Rattled, the Lady races back to rustle through countless pill bottles. There are two types of morphine. One is immediate- (quick) release and one is extended- (slow) release. Today she'll need immediate-release so the Lady grabs the one labeled Morphine ER (**EEEEE**mmediate-release) and gives her one. It's 1 p.m. so she can have another in 12 hours. Four hours later, the Sister calls for more morphine. Hmmm . . . she can't have any this soon. This isn't good but, luckily, she falls back asleep. Six hours later, Donna (who's a registered nurse) questions what morphine was given. It just doesn't sound right—the 12-hour part. The Lady texts back she's got it under control. (But just in case, she has a look at the bottle and, *Heaven have MERCY and Baby Girl forgive us!*, she's given her the WRONG one. The long *E* sound in the word *immediate* made her grab the ER (extended-release—a little bit over a long period of time). She should have given her the IR (immediate-release—fast and every six hours). By 9 p.m., the Sister wakes up to the Lady's face only inches from her own (in the middle of making sure she's still breathing) and wants more morphine. How will she make it another four hours? We have no idea.

You are warned from day one to stay on top of pain management. If it gets out of control, the patient is in trouble. The Sister didn't fail; the Lady did—human error. It makes us ill denying her and we go to bed wracked with guilt. "Dear GOD," the Lady says out loud into the darkness, "I *beg* you to please keep her sleeping until one in the morning and I'll never let this happen again. I *promise!*" I'm not sure if other frogs can even cry, but my eyes tear up as I type this because He heard her.

. . . to be continued. We've gotta go now.

Yours,

Frog

♦　♦　♦　♦　♦　♦　♦　♦

The Frog Letters

FEBRUARY 25, 2011

Dear Family,

(. . . continuation of my previous letter) Friday, the Sister awakens and believes it's Thursday. Believing she was discharged hours after Wednesday's surgery, 24 hours are missing. Any foggy memories of mean nurses are erased! Proclaiming several times that she can't go through this again, she lies for three days, unwilling to move her body but inches at a time, due to pain in her liver. The Lady parades food and drink in front of her, but a bite or sip of either causes unbearable stomach pain. For a while, her urine turns the color of chocolate milk, she runs a fever and gets chills. Shortness of breath is another issue. Over the next week, her morphine doses go from right on time, to some, to none. From lying immobile, her weight rapidly dwindles. She's only pounds away from dipping below 100. The Lady gets tough with her and begins pushing food and drink every two hours, insisting she must eat something, if only a few bites. Replying she doesn't want to waste food, the Lady goes against their upbringing by saying, "Who cares? It's only food. We'll get more!"

On Friday, the Brother returns with a sack in tow—Cheese Nips, pretzels, wafer and animal cookies, and two varieties of chocolate chip cookies. He spends the day sampling what he can, as part of his determination to get his jaw working. He confides he's forgotten how to chew and keeps biting his tongue. Saturday, he wakes and the right side (surgery side) of his face is humongous and disfigured. "Did you break your jaw?" she asks. "We've got to get you to Urgent Care." He refuses and here's the reality of the situation, we're tired and the Sister can't be left alone. If he had agreed, we would have loaded up and driven off. His refusal comes as a relief. Sunday, not much better, the Lady announces we need to take the Brother to the emergency room. Again, he refuses. Days later, his face returns to normal and he begins nibbling lessons again.

You're probably wondering how on earth they go on. I'll tell you in my next letter.

Yours,

Frog

♦　♦　♦　♦　♦　♦　♦　♦

Dear Family,

This is the story of how they go on.
They wake each day and forge ahead because the path this family walks is blessed. Some would say, *BLESSED? What, with this awful journey you describe? You call that blessed?* There's no mistaking it, blessed they are. From those in Texas, to Donna, and to the Mom and Dad, they share their stories with each other. Stories of the people who are placed in their paths, unspoken needs that are met, and prayers that are answered. This happens so often, some may chalk it up to coincidence. Some may call it lucky, but we see it for what it is—blessed.

The following are just some of their **Random Blessings**:

~ Random Blessing: A card from the Dad arrived in the mail for the Lady. Shiny dimes spilled onto her lap, revealing the collection he had found. Then, the Sister drove to the park before the sun had even risen. After walking the trails, she approached the car. For a millisecond, something flashed on the ground catching her eye. Reaching down to see what it was, she picked up a shiny dime—a dime she wouldn't normally have been able to see in darkness. I wonder, are *you* finding dimes?

~ Random Blessing: Remember the time the Lady's heart was troubled over information withheld from the Sister? And how she wanted to find that one person who could tell her it was going to be okay? Cecelia and the Lady were friends in elementary school. She had a younger sister, Beth, the same age as the Sister. They, too, were friends. Their families attended church together. On the very day I sent you that letter, an e-mail arrived from Cecelia, the only person in the Lady's life (that she knows of) who's walked in her shoes. Someone who had spent all those unknown hours and countless days while months flipped by on the calendar—her sister's shadow as she watched Beth lose her battle with cancer. Cecelia is one who knows what it feels like to stare, stare, stare (eternity!) into the eyes of her baby sister and see for herself those words you hear with your eyes. At one time, she was faced with the same type of decisions the Lady is facing. She reveals scenes that hit our hearts like nails and make us feel her pain. Cecelia told the Lady, "Beth told me she was scared and looked at me. I said 'Me too,' folded my arms across my chest and backed up against the wall . . . " Now, she sends the Lady words of comfort, telling her what she needs to hear, freeing her from the emotional bondage of a secret. (By the way, Cecelia found a dime in an odd location of her laundry room yesterday.)

~ Random Blessing: Being forewarned by the dealership that the 30,000-mile service on her car was going to be a BIG one, a couple months in advance, the Lady decides to find out their definition of *big* and calls to ask. "Now let's go back to where you said the word *big*. Like, what exactly are we talking? (pause) Really? $599.00?" Hanging up the phone, the Lady immediately said a prayer telling God she can't be worried about this right now so she's passing it on to Him to handle. She never told another soul about this except me. It wasn't long before a monetary gift arrived from their Uncle Jim in Colorado. Someone told him to send help, and it certainly wasn't either one of us! When we still had plenty of time before it needed that "big" service, one Sunday, the Lady and I went to put gas in the car while it was still dark outside. The Check Engine light came on. It seemed so mean and threatening as it glared at us in the darkened interior. Later, en route to church with the Sister, the Lady was telling her about the indicator light. Still driving, she started saying a prayer out loud telling Him to turn off that light and take that worry from her. Furthermore, she wasn't going to give it another thought and would consider it done! Granted, after parking at church, she was just a teeny bit disappointed it was still shining but, with conviction and faith, once again she said, "I'm giving this up to You!" After church, as we left the parking lot, the Lady told us to have a look. The Check Engine light was off.

~ Random Blessing: A couple weeks later, the Lady was in the dentist chair talking with Dr. Glover about the Check Engine light story. "Yes! He just keeps taking care of us!" The Lady left Dr. Glover's office. About 10 miles out of town, in Joshua, the car had a complete power failure. Crossing a lane of traffic on momentum alone, we reached the shoulder of the road and continued to coast right up to the door of Kurt's Off-Road Automotive and Diesel Repair Center. What a blessing it was because He didn't leave us stranded in the far lane or on a back road. He dropped us at a safe place with a mechanic. Kurt hooked the car up to a machine to get an idea what was wrong with it, took it for a short spin, when the Check Engine light went off.

"What do I owe you?" the Lady asked.

"Nah, don't worry about it. I got you covered. (That sounded incredibly Biblical at the time.) Hopefully, you'll make it home," Kurt said.

(Warning! This is going to be a long letter! In my defense, I haven't written in a week. Now, where was I? Oh yeah . . .)

~ Random Blessing: There was the time we went to Subway and the woman behind the counter, noticing the patient bracelet on the Sister's wrist, asked if she'd just been released from the hospital. When the Sister told her she had cancer and just had treatment, the woman said, "Oh my gosh, Sweetheart! Can I come and give you a hug?" She did just that and then she said, "I'll be thinking about you!" Such simple gestures of compassion aren't forgotten by us. Last week, when the Lady and I entered Subway and ordered a six-inch ham and cheese on wheat, the Lady told the young man behind the counter, "This is a very important sandwich you're making. My sister lost 11½ lbs. in a week because of cancer treatment to her liver. She wants Subway so. . . here I am!" The Lady noticed a second (unasked for) layer of ham was added to the sandwich. There was a kindness in this person who stood before us in this particular Subway on this particular day. He talked so freely with us, strangers that we were. At the time, I couldn't help but feel there was more to this than a casual meeting. We weren't standing face-to-face talking right then, that minute, for no reason. He was placed in our path.

~ Random Blessing: Then there was the time it took the Lady and me hours to get the Sister's prescription filled. When we arrived home, the Sister quietly said she didn't want to take that medicine after all. "Are you mad at me?" she asked. The Lady looked down at the Sister lying on the couch, having a bad day, and told her she can't think of a single thing that the Sister could do that would make her mad. As we start to leave the room, we almost miss hearing her say, "I love you . . . but you know that already, right?" Taking a couple of steps back in her direction, the Lady replies, "Yes, (what a blessing!) I know that."

~ Random Blessing: Sometimes we hear words from others that strike at just the right moment. A group e-mail was forwarded from Tina (Fellowship Valley) and, in the midst of all those words, the beacon that falls on the words meant for us: *Before they call, I will answer... (Isaiah 65:24).* Another example was a recent e-mail from Cecelia. She wrote, *I feel like you and I are now sisters, not only in Christ, but also in a club that nobody really wants to join. We've had this membership thrust upon us and have had to live it out. It's like when we found out that our Nicholas had muscular dystrophy—we walked through a doorway, and the door closed behind us. There's no way to go back through it to take another path, we just have to go on. These are your wilderness days. I pray that your wandering ends in a beautiful place.*

(Ok, I'm almost done. I promise I'm wrapping up this letter.)

~ Random Blessing: Today, we headed back to Dr. Glover's office. There was some sort of reduction thing going on when the Lady's charges were calculated. She questions Dana, and Dana says, "Nope, that's what I was told to charge!" When Dr. Glover appears, the Lady gives him a hug and thanks him. He says, "That's for living a clean life!"

~ Random Blessing: Stopping back by Kurt's Off-Road Automotive and Diesel Repair Center, in Joshua, we catch Kurt in his office, sitting behind his desk. He shares a piece of his life with us. His brother died last April, and his Mom took it very hard. These words are still hard for him, and he struggles to say them. Tears surface in his eyes as he continues. In her sorrow one day, his Mom went to the cemetery to visit. As she was leaving the cemetery, sliding back behind the wheel of the car, the antenna on the hood of the car started waving back and forth in an exaggerated manner. It was a clear day with no wind. There were no trees in the area where something could've fallen, triggering the movement. Her eyes, being drawn to the antenna, witnessed a lone butterfly fly past. She felt it was a sign from her son. (At that moment, it reminded me of the Sister because she *too* speaks of butterflies. Hmmm . . . odd. He could've told any story, but he chose to tell us one that makes us think of the Sister.)

We thanked Kurt for helping us the other day and for his kindness.

He said, "I live my life helping others. That's why I'll never be rich!" We laugh. "But, life's not about me." These were his exact words. Where have you heard *those* before? "I have to look in the mirror when I get up in the morning. I have to live with myself and it's a good feeling when I don't have to worry about my conscience."

What more could I possibly add to this? I guess the Sister says it best, "God's constantly saying to us, 'I'm there! I'm there! I'm there!'"

(Cracking my knuckles . . .) I rest my case.

Yours,

Frog

◆   ◆   ◆   ◆   ◆   ◆   ◆   ◆

MARCH 4, 2011

Dear Family,

The Sister's memories have turned sentimental lately. She says, "Ask Dad if he'll bring me a shark's tooth from his collection when he comes. I remember how much he loves his arrowheads and shark teeth." (A small box of artifacts, family treasures really, arrive for her in the mail from the Dad.) The Sister says, "You know that fancy glass bottle in my bathroom? That Brogdon boy gave it to me back in elementary school. It used to have liquid bath soap in it and I thought the jar was so pretty I kept it even though it was empty." (Each memory brings another with it.) "When I was really young," the Sister says, "Mom and Dad got me a necklace for Christmas one year. It was in the shape of a tiny Bible with a small little diamond on the outside."

"Heeeey," the Lady interrupts, "I remember that!"

The Sister continues, "And you could open it and there was a place for two little pictures."

"Only it was really too small for pictures, right?"

The Sister said, "Yeah. I kept it for a long time, until I was an adult, then lost it somehow. The last time I saw it, Mom and I were at a store and she found it in the pocket of her coat! I don't know what happened to it after that. That's always bothered me. I wish I still had it."

Yours,

Frog

♦ ♦ ♦ ♦ ♦ ♦ ♦ ♦

MARCH 8, 2011

Dear Family,

The Lady said something's been bothering her; I need to address it and tell you the truth of the matter. Remember last week when Dr. Glover hugged her then said, *"That's for livin' a clean life?"* Something about that statement has bothered her. She wonders if anyone else ever feels the same way at times. It's like when someone says, "You're so *sweet!*" The first thing you think of is all the rottenness about you that no one except God knows about. You know—all the times you direct your life, fail to make the right decision, have a mean thought, are lazy, don't witness to another. The secrets you guard from others, the *real* you—the part of you you're not proud of. Do you ever feel like that?

The Lady wants you to know that being a Christian isn't easy. The Lady works at it every single day and fights her battles against sin by trying to make right decisions and scouring the Bible to find answers on how she should live. Issues come up all the time—part of just trying to live in this world. Sure, she has some good traits but, quite frankly, she's a work in progress. She's human.

After her appointment with Dr. Glover, the Lady got a random group e-mail from Renee's parents that seemed to sum it up. She wants me to share it with you because it makes perfect sense and is wonderfully worded:

WHEN I SAY, "I AM A CHRISTIAN"

When I say, "I am a Christian"
I'm not shouting, "I've been saved!"
I'm whispering, "I get lost!
That's why I chose this way"
When I say, "I am a Christian"
I don't speak with human pride
I'm confessing that I stumble—

Needing God to be my guide
When I say, "I am a Christian"
I'm not trying to be strong
I'm professing that I'm weak
And pray for strength to carry on
When I say, "I am a Christian"
I'm not bragging of success
I'm admitting that I've failed
And cannot ever pay the debt
When I say, "I am a Christian"
I don't think I know it all
I submit to my confusion
Asking humbly to be taught
When I say, "I am a Christian"
I'm not claiming to be perfect
My flaws are all too visible
But God believes I'm worth it
When I say, "I am a Christian"
I still feel the sting of pain
I have my share of heartache,
Which is why I seek His name
When I say, "I am a Christian"
I do not wish to judge
I have no authority . . .
I only know I'm loved

(Used by Permission - Copyright 1988 Carol Wimmer)

Last Sunday, in North Carolina, was Women's Sunday at the
Parents' church. The Mom was asked to speak to everyone about how
God's been there for this family. She's one of the few within this clan
who is confident at public speaking. The family considers shyness a
hereditary gene passed down from the Dad to various children and
grandchildren. The Sister is the most afflicted. For instance, in an
attempt to draw attention away from herself and avoid cashier small-
talk, she used to pass money to another sibling to pay for her purchases
as they approached the cash register. As an adult, she relishes the
quiet, privacy of her home and life, perfectly content to let others
be social butterflies—never feeling the need, nor wanting, to be the
center of attention.

The Lady used to hyperventilate in school, fearing she'd be asked a question by the teacher or asked to read aloud. Her face would burn red-hot! She opened up more when she reached 40 and realized half the population was now younger than herself. She remembered when she was a kid how she categorized all older adults as wise, mature, and having it all together. She figured the younger generation would make that same assumption about her and, for some ridiculous reason, it made her braver in this world.

The Lady's not a public speaker, though, and that's one thing she wishes she could do. Then maybe, by some great fortune from above, she'd be asked to tour for a year with The Women of Faith as a speaker. (The Mom and the Lady love attending those conferences.) Those speakers are polished, funny, and perfect in telling great stories. The Lady said she'd be the one speaker the women could relate to most. She would get up on the stage (makeup not quite right and hair in need of a major overhaul) and begin telling her own stories. She'd tell them about her failures (as much as time allows) or confess a story about how she really stinks at this or that and how God helps her straighten her life out, again, every day. The women would listen and know exactly what she was talking about, nodding to those around them in agreement, and think, "I totally stink like that *too*! Finally, someone who's admitting it out loud!" Because she was completely healed, sometimes the Sister would travel with the Lady and, when the crowd finds out about her cancer journey, they would chant, "SISTER! SISTER! SISTER!" The Sister would agree to cross the stage and wave to everyone as long as she didn't have to speak, and the Lady would walk beside her, and they wouldn't loiter.

Recently, the Sister's been thinking about heaven a lot and when she sees herself in heaven she said everyone's singing and dancing in praise. But when she sees herself, she's standing right next to Jesus and she's not dancing or singing out loud because she's so shy. She's singing and dancing in her heart. "Do you think He'll understand?" the Sister asks. *Oh my precious sister!* the Lady thinks. While relaying this story to the crowds at the conferences, the Lady won't be polished about it. No, she'll choke up when she speaks. Her face will get blotchy red and her nose will run profusely. Even *now* she chokes up whenever she speaks of her sister. The women will think, *Yes! I understand. I love my sister TOO!* as they rummage in their purses for a tissue.

Maybe smaller groups are more in her future. Maybe she'll tell stories around the campfire at Fellowship Valley. Propping one foot on a small boulder and resting her elbow across her knee, she'll roast a marshmallow until it flames up, eating the charred shell and re-roasting the rest. She'll gaze at the top of the tree line of the tall Georgia pines with a faraway look in her eye. Then she'll grab everyone's attention in amazement as she starts with, "My closest companion for a while was a frog yard ornament." Instead of closing the night by holding hands in a circle and singing *Kum-ba-ya*, they'll break out singing *Lifesong* by Casting Crowns with their arms raised in a dance.

Maybe she'll heed Ron's (her church friend from where she used to live) advice when he recently told her she could make practically a small fortune in tips if she were their beer cart girl at the golf coarse. "You wanna a beer?" she'd ask. "Sure! No problem. But *first* you'll have to pass a test." Then she'd quickly produce two small, plastic cups—the kind in which meds are delivered in retirement homes. "A taste test! Now, close your eyes. Which one do you like best? Sample A or Sample B?" Results are revealed at the Pro Shop that nine out of ten golfers chose Sample B, which just so happened to be Mountain Dew! After repainting the cart a bold green color, the Lady would now become (practically a hero in their eyes for making them see the light) their new Mountain Dew cart girl! Yet, making her feel only *slightly* better about her career choice, all the while seriously questioning herself. Was she sure she stayed on the right path and it led here (as she surveys the cart with slight disdain now) or was this the direct result of her taking over the steering wheel of her life, once again?

Maybe her voice won't even be heard. Perhaps the world will hear her through me and my letters home. Regardless, I do know that wherever she ends up, or whatever she ends up doing, it'll be by following the path He chose for her. (Plus, after that possible cart scenario, she's more determined than ever!)

As for me, perhaps I'll develop an insatiable desire to take up knitting and join a group that meets every Thursday night at 7 p.m. You can reveal tales about me as everyone rocks back and forth in chairs listening, as our harmonious needles click a mile a minute.

Yours,

Frog

♦　♦　♦　♦　♦　♦　♦　♦

MARCH 12, 2011

Dear Family,

   The Sister didn't leave the house for three weeks after chemoembolization to her liver—until she was forced to do so. A voice message was left on the answering machine telling her to be at the cancer center Wednesday morning. I'm not going to lie to you, she took a beating having that procedure and said if she'd known in advance how bad it was going to be, well, she wouldn't have done it!
   She's not back to normal yet. For a while, she said she felt anxious and we could tell by the way she said it. This was a code for politely saying go away and leave me alone. We were annoying to her in our constant hovering and appearances to see if she wanted something to eat or wanted her blanket heated in the dryer. Even now, she'll get up in the morning, straighten her blanket while gasping for breath, and wish she could collapse back on the couch. Outside of getting dressed, and an occasional stop in the kitchen, she's sitting up or lying down on the couch all day. This goes beyond tired; it's absolute fatigue. (They told me before the Sister got sick last April, she was very energetic and active.) Signs of no energy appear in actions and routines that seem entirely off-kilter. Her bath towel, always folded with Army precision in the past, is haphazardly thrown across the shower door to dry. Small piles appear, on the table next to her or the floor beside her, bearing empty wrappers of candy, cheese, popsicles, and cookies. Used bowls and cups never make it further than an arm's length away before coming to rest, their contents left to harden and dry until the Lady catches sight of them and gathers everything up to set things straight again.
   The pain is still with her but not to the extent it was the first two weeks after that procedure. Refusing any pain medication, she fears addiction and doesn't want to battle *that* once she gets through with cancer. Waves of nausea assail her, so the Lady tells her it's the toxins from the tumors. "They're dying!" she proclaims, with hope

the Sister will think, *Yes! They're dying so now I can feel good about being sick because it means I'm getting well!* The coming and going of feeling in her fingertips and toes has stopped because now she can't feel them at all. The Sister struggles to hold a pen to write.

Trying to bring some sort of hope to the Sister, the Lady reads words of inspiration, only to get a response such as, *That's easy to say when you're not sick.* True words, I'm sure. However, this isn't the Sister I know and it reminds me of the times she was so ill during chemo treatments that she didn't want to listen to her favorite songs as we drove down the road. This must be the breaking point a person comes to when living with constant sickness for a long time.

Sunday, we sat between Linda and Janet before the church service began. Linda, whenever I see her, reminds me of a whisper. I don't know why because I'm not referring to her speech, but her size. She's a tiny, sweet woman who's filled with so much power in what she says. She speaks the right words to the Lady. The Lady always seeks her out wherever we sit. She lends a shoulder if the Lady just needs a quick cry. On this day, the women were gabbing about makeup tips. We told them it doesn't matter how sick the Sister is, that's one thing she does every day—puts on her makeup.

Since this church started a series on healing, we desperately wished all the Lady's family were sitting with us. The pastor asked anyone who was sick and needed prayer to stand. The Lady stood. Having told no one this except Ron (from her old church) and her Uncle Jim, in August when the Lady had her yearly exam, we had to go back the following week to have her blood tests redone. The readings were off and they wanted to double check them. The following week we returned and her doctor, knowing what her recent lifestyle involved, said this could very well be stress-related.

Getting back to the story . . . so she stood up and the pastor said, "If you have a heart condition or diabetes," then in the same breath he said, "liver cancer (baby Sister)." It was as if God were speaking to us and saying pay attention! She could feel Janet and Linda stand at her side and place a hand on her back in prayer support. Immediately, it felt like every care in the world that was hampering her well-being was instantly removed. Her whole insides felt cleansed or erased. That's the only way she could describe it. She breathed better than she could ever remember and felt 10 years younger. She turned to

Linda and said, "I feel fabulous!" It wasn't just her because later, Linda said, "I just really felt like the Lord touched us both . . . "

We drove home feeling all "Zippity Doo Dah-ish," took one look at the Brother and Sister, and didn't have the guts to tell them the Lady was feeling nothing short of incredible! Looking at the siblings, we told them about the sermons on healing that were coming up and how next Sunday we all needed to go—all of us.

Yours,

Frog

~ Random Blessing: Linda turned to the Lady and said she felt led to pay for anything the Sister wanted from the Avon catalog. Linda said, "It'll make her feel nice to have some new makeup. She can pick out anything she wants." The Lady tells her that's really not necessary, God has been providing for them. Then she laughs when it dawns on her that it's people exactly *like* Linda who are the providers! It wasn't until we were driving home that I reminded the Lady, didn't she remember just a couple days ago the Sister was reminiscing about when they were growing up and how the Mom used Avon's *Skin So Soft*? The Sister always loved the smell of it. She should tell Linda if she wants to give the Sister another memory to touch her heart, *Skin So Soft* will work. It's perfect!

♦ ♦ ♦ ♦ ♦ ♦ ♦ ♦

MARCH 16, 2011

Dear Family,

For reasons I don't understand, I find it unbelievably difficult to write to you about the Dad. Perhaps it's because he's so many states away and I can't see everything firsthand to accurately report back to you. I'll do a quick report on him to bring you up-to-date.

After his eight-day hospitalization in August, due to the side effects from the Zometa IV treatment for his bones, the Dad's recovery was slow. On the first of September, he confided to the Lady that he was worried. Unable to eat since nothing smelled or tasted good to him, he dropped 24 pounds. In desperation, the Mom paraded his favorite dishes before him and made mad dashes, near and far, to retrieve "food love offerings" for him. These all resulted in failed attempts that we recognize ourselves.

Because of the reaction the Dad had to Zometa, that drug wasn't given to him again for five months, and then in smaller doses. His treatment over the next six months consisted of one Revlimid pill a day for 21 straight days, a one- or two-week break, then another round of pills began. You might think, *What luck! Only one pill a day!* However, that was not the case. Overall, whether due to the drugs or cancer, he suffered from pain under his ribs, abdominal pain, low energy, slow heart rate, low blood pressure, circulation problems, and kidney pain that caused pain with each breath. Blood clots developed causing his legs and feet to swell to a ginormous size. Walking became so difficult he walked like he was crippled. Travel by plane or car, for any length time, was banned because of clots. He was prescribed Coumadin but, after one pill, he started spitting up blood for several days. He was instructed not to lift anything over five pounds or his bones could break. When a person has bone cancer, bones cannot be repaired. With that news, his lifetime hobby of golfing ceased.

Because the Parents' bed sits so high, he was unable to comfortably maneuver getting in and out of bed without having immense pain

---

The Frog Letters

in the formerly tumored arm. His lounge chair in the living room became his spot both day and night. That arrangement hasn't changed in eight months. The Mom, sitting or lying on the couch next to him, keeps her vigil over him. If he rises in the middle of the night, she gets up, makes her way in the dark to stand in the distance, and watches over him until they are both safely back in their new night spots. That reminds me of the Lady, as she watches over the Sister. The Dad tells us, every night before he goes to sleep, he rests his elbow on the chair's armrest then raises his palm toward the sky and says a prayer over his kids in Texas. The Sister and Lady love hearing that story. It touches their hearts.

By November, he's still trying to make his way through the treatments. He said with each day that goes by, with each pill taken, a little more energy is taken away. He watches the calendar, marking his three-week progress of daily pills, waiting and willing day number 21 to hurry and arrive so the break between treatments can begin. During breaks, he tries to recover as much as possible before the next round begins. Sounds so familiar, huh?

His siblings and friends will travel from one coast to the other to reassure themselves of his safety. They love him. People love him. He's a lovable man. The Mom will incorporate a set of new rules designed for these visitors. If the Dad needs a nap, it's declared everyone in attendance must take a nap too. Her brothers-in-law laugh as they recall their forced naps, but she takes her caregiving very seriously, and they admire and love her for that. Each of his siblings are very much aware of the inner struggle the Dad battles, a battle he relates not only to them, but to the people at his church and his doctors. He simply can't move past it, and it takes on an urgency of near desperation. He's got to get back to Texas and check on his kids!

Both households are literally stuck. He's unable to travel and we're unable to travel. It's been really quite heart-wrenching hearing of the numerous failed attempts to schedule a trip, but the doctors say he'd never make it here and back. Both the Lady's oldest son, Kyle, and the Dad's brother, Jim, in Colorado, offer to drive the Parents to Texas. However, with the blood clots, the Dad couldn't travel that far unless they stopped every 30 minutes and let him walk around. At that rate, the trip would be unbearable! So, Jim did the next best thing. In December, he brought the Parents and the siblings together by sending a webcam to each household.

On February 1, 2011, blood tests showed the Dad's cancer was in remission. Once he gained strength, he was cleared for travel. So, there you have it; the Dad's story has been updated.

Yours,

Frog

♦ ♦ ♦ ♦ ♦ ♦ ♦ ♦

MARCH 22, 2011

Dear Family,

Once, someone told me she couldn't bear to read my letters home to you any more. It got her down too much. I spent time wondering if maybe this was also the case with you. Maybe I should steer away from the parts of their lives that make people feel uncomfortable. However, I know in my heart I'm not supposed to do that—just tell half the story, the good parts—leaving out the struggles. The whole idea is just too unrealistic of life. The struggles are needed to recognize and appreciate the joys and to grow. I hope you're with me on this, so here we go.

Thursday, at 8:30 a.m. in radiation, the Sister is having CT scans taken of her liver to see if the chemoembolization procedure worked. At the same time, a few doors down, the Brother is in a room being told they're considering putting a permanent feeding tube in his stomach. The one he sports now, of temporary quality, has been used daily for 13 months. He leaves with mixed emotions about what this could really imply.

Saturday morning, the Lady and I ran to get groceries. When we got back, a while later, we noticed the Sister wasn't around. She was in the back of the house in her bathroom. Knocking on the door, the Lady asked if she was okay. It took a while but, eventually, the Sister said she was fine. When a couple hours went by and she still hadn't made an appearance, we went back again and started knocking. She didn't answer. I thought the Sister probably passed out because she doesn't have any energy, but I peeked through the one-inch space under the door and told the Lady I could see her feet. Knocking harder, the Lady said if she needed some help, to answer her. The Sister said she'd be out in a while, she was fine, but that was said in her crying voice.

We started watching the clock and didn't like this one bit. A couple more hours passed before the Lady looked under the door. There were no feet this time, which means the Sister was in her closet. Remember how awful it was the other time this happened?

"Honey, open the door and let me in! Can you hear me? (Sister's name), open UP!"

Still in her crying voice, "I don't feel good. I'll be out soon."

We don't believe her anymore. Something's desperately wrong and we become anxious.

"Please come out. I just want to be with you. Just . . . just whatever it is, I can help you. We can pray together," the Lady pleaded.

She promised again, "In a little bit."

Six hours passed since her disappearance. For six hours, she stayed in solitude. Then she came out to take her place on the couch to fall asleep. We wanted to shake her awake and ask, *What just happened? You must say!* However, once we looked at her, curled up on her side and sleeping, we let all the anxiety of the day be released. We have to believe whatever internal battle she had just fought, she had also won.

Over the course of several weeks, the Sister asked, "Will you find that one verse and read it to me again?" Flipping pages, the Lady stops to read, "Is anyone among you sick? Let them call the elders of the church to pray over them and anoint them with oil in the name of the Lord."

The Sister asks, "Is that in the Old or New Testament?"

"New, James 5:14."

The Sister is hung up on this verse. It speaks deeply to her. Only the three of us have knowledge of this. No, make that four . . .

Cleared for travel, the Dad and Mom journey to see their children. It was a slow one because of his condition. On Sunday, my wish from last week becomes reality. The family attends church together as a unit bonded by blood and by belief. After praise with music, there was a time for prayer before the service began. The elders and deacons of the church stood up front to pray over any special needs. Linda came to the Sister, took her hand in hers, and with faith and trust (not only in God but in the small woman who now stands before her), the Sister stood and walked with Linda over to the pastor. The rest of the family followed closely behind. They stood in a circle with hands joined, as the pastor anointed the Sister with oil and then prayed a prayer of healing over her. The second they settled back into their seats, unable to contain her joy, she told the Lady he anointed her with oil! God, the fourth and only other one to know, met her desire.

Monday morning, the Lady and Mom browsed through the LifeWay store. Almost crossing the threshold to exit, the Lady looked down and exclaimed to all in the vicinity to look! Gaining attention from a few, she reached down, picked up a shiny dime, and excitedly let them know in their family this means God is with them! They would surely need this reminder because three hours later, the Mom, Sister, Lady, and I found ourselves in a room at the cancer center with Dr. Choufani as he told us the CT scan results revealed the chemoembolization did not work on the liver tumors. Driving home, we joked about how the scans needed to be retaken. The ones they had were old news now that the Sister was anointed and healed, but the Lady's eyes couldn't hide her sorrowful heart. Believe me, it has nothing to do with lack of faith for a healing, but everything to do with what we saw the Sister endure this past month—the incredible pain, suffering, loss of weight, energy, and breath. Surely even the *least* hopeful person would expect more than nothing for all that.

We dropped the Mom off at the hotel, drove home, and the Sister sat down on the couch to read a book. We could see the back of her head as the Lady ironed in the kitchen. Not really thinking of anything as she tackled her task, loud words entered her mind full-force, strong, with a sense of urgency. Not pondering over the words, nor wasting a second, she yelled the Sister's name and boldly repeats them, "(For) we live by faith, not by sight!" (2 Corinthians 5:7) The Sister told us she was reading her book when her mind had just started to think about what Dr. Choufani told us but, within a split second, the Lady yelled those words at her. We were all amazed and really felt blessed. (I'm there!)

A bounty of gifts have been bestowed on this family that they consider to be heaven-sent, believing God places on the hearts of others to show His love through them. Linda brought a gift sack to church for the Sister filled with an assortment of Avon products to make her feel special, including her Skin So Soft memory. A nice ceramic plaque with a frog on it arrives (via the Parents) from Sue, the secretary for their church. It reads, *John 3:16 - You Are Loved.* Sue has experienced her own grief in life by losing her sixteen-year-old daughter, who collapsed while running due to an unknown heart condition. She is also a breast cancer survivor. Never having met the siblings, Sue reminds the Parents to make sure they let their kids know she cares about each one of them. The Mom and Dad, thinking of my family, produce a red gift box for you.

Yours,

Frog

♦ ♦ ♦ ♦ ♦ ♦ ♦ ♦

MARCH 25, 2011

Dear Family,

Spending the rest of the week with the Parents was great! For lunch on Tuesday, we all met in Mansfield, at Our Place, with Ken and Lu Ella. Any time spent with these people is great! (I don't want to turn into a "restaurant reviewer frog-person," but this restaurant is always packed for a reason. The food is good, the servings are large, and they have a huge list of homemade pies from which to choose.)

During the week, the Parents had a chance to meet a lot of people featured in my letters home. The Dad met Dr. Choufani. They dropped off the Lady's late birthday card to Raymond at JPS hospital. They met the Clown (Yes, even him!), and Kurt from Kurt's Off-Road Automotive and Diesel Repair Center. They saw the God's Heart gate and supported the Relay For Life drive at the cancer center.

Time was spent in private conversations. The Sister asked the Parents to please forgive all the wrongs she'd done as a kid. She feels badly about a lot of things, but the Parents told her not to worry. They love her so much and are proud of the person she is today. The Mom confides, regularly she climbs the stairs in their home to spend time in the Lady's former bedroom. It makes her feel close to the Lady when she does this. While there, she'll pray for her children in Texas. The Dad told the Sister things in his past that he's accomplished that none of his kids know about because he's quiet about stuff like that. The Sister, told a story of how every day when she was in elementary school she'd get up and declare *that* day was the day she wasn't going to do anything wrong. She'd watch every thought, every word, and every action. Then every night, she realized at some point during the day she'd failed again.

You must be wondering about the results from the Sister's anointing that Sunday. Immediately after the service, I asked how she was feeling. Not to be "greedy" for an instant healing, but maybe so. Ha! What? I love her! Who wouldn't? The rest of Sunday and

Monday morning, the top middle of her chest was hurting like never before. The Lady was telling her it's the healing! Claim it! It was a little discouraging on Monday when Dr. Choufani said the chemoembolization did nothing for the liver tumors, but Linda (from church) said the most remarkable thing. Now no one can dispute her healing was from God. That really makes perfect sense. Monday, all of us noticed little changes beginning in the Sister. For starters, her energy level rose above zero. She began to eat. Her breathing was improving. Within a couple of days, she went to the movies and ate popcorn with the Mom.

On Thursday, Donna flew in from New Jersey. Since the Parents and Donna live out of state, they wanted to see the cemetery. All of us walked around the cemetery where the Sister had picked out her spot all those many months ago and it wasn't even a sad affair. She wasn't on her deathbed and she had energy so we walked and walked all over the cemetery.

Friday was the Parents' 55th wedding anniversary. The Lady and I headed over to pick up the cake she'd ordered to take to the restaurant before we all met for dinner. The bakery lady was so happy when we arrived. She said she'd told all her staff what was piped in frosting around the outside of the cake platter. She loved it so much! That night at the restaurant, Donna had tears in her eyes after getting up to look at the cake.

So she became his wife, and he loved her . . . Genesis 24:67

Yours,

Frog

◆　◆　◆　◆　◆　◆　◆　◆

MARCH 31, 2011

Dear Family,

The Sister got a call from Lou last week. She's one of Dr. Choufani's chemo nurses we love so much. She said it was time to begin a new treatment and she needed us to stop in sometime before April 4th to pick up the paperwork. The Lady and I made a trip to the cancer center this week to pick up the papers.

We sat in the partially-filled room waiting for Lou. Taking a seat next to us, she explained information about the next drug they will use for treatment and the possible side effects involved. The Sister will now begin what they consider the second level of cancer care. This means the best drug for her type cancer has already been used and is no longer effective. Anything they try from here on out will be inferior to what she's previously been given, but they always hope to get a positive response. Depending on the side effects, they may switch the drugs from time to time to see what kind of reaction she has. We should be aware there's always the possibility the side effects may cause her to decide to stop treatment, if it comes down to her quality of life.

The level after this will be her final care. We didn't know there were actual *levels* of care. Second level sounded so much more friendlier until it turned into the level just before final care. That is, unless final care means the person is healed and good to go. On that note, the Lady looks at all the people sitting among us. Who's approaching final care in this room and doesn't even know it? The Lady's heart turns so heavy with the thought, she interrupts, "I think I'm going to start crying." Lou says, "Oh no! I think I'm going to start crying, too!" We follow her to a private room.

"This is the time we tell patients to get their business in order."

"We have her will done. Her plot is nearly paid for."

"What about a Medical Power of Attorney?"

"Yes . . ."

DianaRae   161

"Forms to decline life support or resuscitate, if that's what she wants?"

"Yes, I think . . . "

"We'll have her sign those on the 4th before she starts treatment. Carry those with you at all times now. Have a copy in her purse. Leave a copy on the refrigerator in case paramedics are ever called and you're not with her. I'm not telling you this because anything's going to happen soon, but my best friend died last month and she was only 51. I was visiting her when it happened. It was her heart."

"Did you take charge with your medical training kicking in?"

"I started CPR and chest compressions on her until the paramedics arrived. I was a mess. Her husband was with me, but I was screaming the whole time."

We grabbed a tissue off the table in front of us and started dabbing our eyes. Like I said before—everyone has a story.

We left the building and made our way through the parking lot, with paperwork blowing in the breeze, knowing full well the conversation we just had with Lou will never reach the Sister's ears.

"Yipes! I didn't like the sound of all that talk," I told the Lady.

"Well," she said, "let's not even think about it, okay? We're lucky. We're believing in the supernatural approach. We're standing firm that she's healed. We're expecting the miracle so, like Linda said, now no one can dispute it. Her healing will be by God's hand."

Yours,

Frog

♦　♦　♦　♦　♦　♦　♦　♦

APRIL 1, 2011

Dear Family,

I have to tell you what happened a couple of days ago. The Sister was sitting in the living room while the Lady was cleaning out her purse at the kitchen table. All of a sudden, the Lady was filled with this incredibly, wonderful gladness in her heart so she said, "Oh my gosh, (Sister's name)! God is *surely* good!" The Sister asked, Why? What happened? The Lady told her nothing happened, she was just feeling it. Right then, she went to check her e-mails and she'd gotten one from Lu Ella three minutes earlier that read:

"Dear Lord, I am lifting (Lady's name) up to you right now. Your comfort is hers right now from your throne. Send it down now precious Lord for her to receive. It is yours now, (Lady's name)! Breathe out the bad and breathe in the good of the Spirit to give His life in your inner being! Take up the joy of the Lord now to minister to your heart and mind! We love you so much and are here for you."

Isn't that amazing?

The Brother found out he's going to be a grandpa for the first time. Having a decent break between his next scheduled office visits, he drove out of state to spend time with his daughter.

The Lady, not having seen her own daughter, Miranda, in two years, planned a quick three-day trip before the Sister started her next treatment. I got to go with her! This was my first time to ever fly on a plane.

Before we boarded the plane, the First Class flight attendants said they'd heard I was going to be on this flight and were glad to meet me. The flight was kind of long so the Lady worked crosswords and read a book about angels while I looked out the window and wondered when the drink and snack cart would come down the aisle. The male flight attendant was so nice when he saw us, he said, "It's a pleasure having you fly with American Airlines today!"

We arrived safely at LAX airport in Los Angeles. We're coming

---

DianaRae

home late Sunday so don't worry about me. I'll let you know when we get back and I'll bring you a souvenir.

Yours,

Frog

♦ ♦ ♦ ♦ ♦ ♦ ♦ ♦

Dear Family,

Okay, we made it back home late last night and had a really fun time! Since the Lady lived in California when she was in high school, there weren't many things she wanted to see. She pretty much left plans up to me since I've never been to California. I really like where Miranda lives. I definitely wanted to see the Hollywood sign and I wanted to see the Hollywood Walk of Fame to see if I could find my favorite frog's star. That's where I found the T-shirt I sent to you.

On Sunday morning, Miranda and her boyfriend, Jon, took us out to eat breakfast in Studio City at Aroma Coffee & Tea Company. It's a really neat outdoor cafe where people can bring their pets with them. It was very different having large and small dogs sitting around us as we ate, but I didn't mind. Before we knew it, it was time to head to the airport and make our way home. I feel so lucky to have made this trip!

Yours,

Frog

♦   ♦   ♦   ♦   ♦   ♦   ♦   ♦

APRIL 8, 2011

Dear Family,

It's Tuesday afternoon. As I begin this letter, I'm sitting on the floor watching both TV and the Sister in equal proportions. With two pillows propped beneath her head, her knees are raised in a conscious attempt to compact herself as she snuggles under two blankets for warmth. There's no chill in the air today. Yesterday, yes, maybe, but today the chill is within her, even though she has no fever. The floor beside her is littered with the TV remote, an unused spit-up bag that will become used within the hour, and a fanny pack. A clear tube line appears between a space in the pack's zipper, snaking up the side of the couch to disappear undercover, continuing a hidden journey to the port in her chest. The chemo pump is dispensing every 30 seconds, right on time. I'm so used to hearing the familiar, constant robotic sound that I continue to hear it, odd as this sounds, even in its absence. She breathes heavily through her mouth with short, quick moans periodically escaping as she sleeps. She is restless.

Monday morning, we made our way to the cancer center, changing the prayer now to one of thanks. Thanks for healing the Sister. The Lady also asked that the really bad side effects of this new drug (the ones that make patients lose their quality of life) not to happen and we would also like to see the Sister's lab results return to normal. There are three readings everyone pays attention to: white blood count (WBC), red blood count (RBC), and hemoglobin (HGB). Some patients' labs, such as the Dad's, will reveal a marker reading from blood work that shows if the cancer is advancing or in remission. The Sister's type of cancer isn't one you can get a marker reading on and we're glad. Marker readings can mess with your emotional well-being if you place value in them. The labs on this day show her WBC has finally creeped just over the line within normal range. We prayed for a normal and we got a normal. None of us can recall the last time anything registered normal so we're happy. Her RBC and HGB have also improved.

Previously, the Sister was on the 24-hour pump Monday through Friday, with the long serious drug treatment on Tuesday, then a three-week break. Her new treatment is different. The new drug will be a long treatment on Monday, with the 24-hour pump Monday through Wednesday, then a one-and-a-half-week break between treatments. The Sister had two pouches drained into her port before the new drug was hooked up. It wasn't long before her eyes started twitching in muscle spasms, then her back, and then her arms. Calling the nurse to come over, she tells her what's happening and the nurse says she'll go speak with the pharmacist. (I never told you this, but yes, there's a pharmacy off the infusion center. It sports a half door so the nurses are frequently going to that door and getting the drugs they need for the patients.) The muscle spasms were very annoying because the Sister had planned to read or watch a movie from a little DVD player Donna had gotten for her. With her eyes twitching, she couldn't do much except sit. Then the spasms started racing around her body. When one seemed to target a muscle by her heart she got scared and called the nurse again. Later, she told us she was afraid not to tell them what was happening because if she died, she didn't want them stumped over what caused it. Now they would know it was those blasted muscle spasms and have a look at her heart.

Sometime in the early hours of morning, the Sister woke up soaked in sweat and piled the blankets on her to ward off chills. By morning, she said she felt like she'd been beaten. She didn't eat this morning; her stomach couldn't take it. It's Wednesday. The pump comes off today. As we pile into the car, the minute the Sister fastens her seat belt, the pump alarm starts sounding—high beep, low beep, high beep, low beep. Removing the machine from the fanny pack, it's indicating that the line is kinked. There are two clasps on the line that can be closed to shut off the flow at a moment's notice. The sisters scramble to check if one clasp accidentally closed the line, which it hadn't. Next, they finger the line from the pump up to the port trying to find the kink. There *is* none so they opt to power the machine down and hope for the best. The best happened—nothing.

It's very early Thursday morning, and as I begin the closure of this letter home, I decide to forsake it for now. I hear gut-retching vomiting coming from the Sister's bathroom. It breaks my heart. I don't feel like writing now.

Today is Friday. All in all, I must say this treatment seemed slightly easier on the body than the one the Sister was on for nine months. Yes, she was sick, chilled, and couldn't eat, but the rotten side effects we were warned about didn't happen. The Sister wants a new wig so today we shopped for one, but she couldn't find one she wanted enough to buy. Afterward, we went to see the movie *Hop*, which was really cute. We went to the first showing because we figured it would be deserted, and it was. The new chemo drug says the Sister shouldn't be around groups of people.

When we returned home, the Sister got her first birthday card in the mail (from her pen pal). She was crying as she handed it to the Lady to read: *Make a Wish on your Birthday . . .* (open card) *. . . and I'll wish it comes true!* (Handwritten message) *You already know God can make all your dreams and wishes come true, you've just got to believe and have faith. I know this to be true, 'cause God blessed me with you! Love, A. O.*

Yours,

Frog

◆   ◆   ◆   ◆   ◆   ◆   ◆   ◆

APRIL 14, 2011

Dear Family,

This was the best week ever! I finally got to see, for the first time, a perfectly healthy Sister. No side effects—none. She had no shortness of breath, liver pain, fatigue, or loss of appetite—no nothing whatsoever! This was a miracle the sisters and I took full advantage of. We went everywhere. You know how the Sister's not supposed to be near groups now? Everywhere we wanted to go, the places appeared nearly deserted. Coincidence? I think not! We saw three movies this week. The Lady took us out to eat at Olive Garden, Saltgrass Steak House, Cici's, and Ol' South Pancake House in Ft. Worth. The Sister gained three pounds this week alone. This means the Sister has now gained back 7 of the 11 ½ pounds she lost back in February. She even mowed a little of the front yard. Can you believe that? Ha! At this rate, I'll be home before you know it.

Remember in my last letter I told you we went looking for a wig and couldn't find anything? When Lu Ella heard about this, she said several weeks ago, the Holy Spirit placed it on her heart to buy the Sister a new wig. She wasn't sure how this would come about, but she knew in God's perfect timing, He would pave the way, which He did!

At the beauty supply store, the Lady and salesclerk began a conversation.

Lady: "Ahhh . . . I love my Sister!"

Salesclerk: "I love my sister too!"

Lady: "But, I *really* love mine!"

Salesclerk: "Me too! I love her!"

No doubt, both women are convinced in the end, they are indeed standing in the presence of another true sister lover! As we browse wigs for the Sister, the store is quiet. We're the only customers. There were lots of wigs there; the entire back wall and four long aisles were filled.

"Okay ladies," the salesclerk said full of good cheer while

DianaRae   169

grabbing a head mannequin in each hand, "Let's go to the fitting room and try on some of these!"

The Sister made her choice known and she looked beautiful. She always does, though. Moments later, the Lady and I left the fitting room to ask the salesclerk, who was busy putting our rejects back in their proper place, if she would take a picture with me and be a part of our cancer journey.

This precious, precious girl looked up from her task and said she'd be honored because she knew exactly what we were feeling. Her sister, the one that she loves, was born with cancer in one eye. She underwent radiation as a baby. "Radiation?" the Lady gasped, trying hard to grasp the concept. Cancer is horrible and mean. It seems there should be an . . . an age limit before you can be afflicted. That was 22 years ago, she continued, and her parents were told to expect mental developmental problems, but that never happened. For having one eye all her life, her sister is a really bright and creative person.

"I think I'll call her right this minute!" the salesclerk said as she pulled a cell phone out of her pocket and began to press in numbers. "I'm going to tell her I've already had a really great morning!"

Yours,

Frog

♦　♦　♦　♦　♦　♦　♦　♦

APRIL 19, 2011

Dear Family,

It's been chemo for the past three days, with the long treatment yesterday. While driving to the center, we thanked God for the lab work that was going to look even better than last time. We thanked Him, in advance, for none of those bad muscle spasms this time! We thanked Him, again, that none of those horrible side effects were going to happen. Her WBC crossed back down to the low side, but her RBC and HGB each rose slightly. The Lady was thinking about quitting her concentration on blood counts now. They are what they are and nitpicking over them every other week could drive a person crazy. Yesterday, with the exception of a few twitches at the beginning of the treatment, there were no out-of-control muscle spasms, and as of this morning, no rotten side effects other than nausea.

This time, we were at the cancer center for six hours. The Lady divided her time between checking on the Sister and satisfying hunger urges. This consisted of walking across the lobby into chemo to ask the Sister what she'd like to eat. Since neither knew what there was to choose from, the Lady walked out of chemo, through the lobby, to the vending room, and wrote a list of everything in the vending machine on a notepad. (She cheated and only wrote *danishes* instead of listing all five varieties offered.) The Lady then walked back through the lobby, and into chemo to let the Sister read the list. After the Sister made her selections, the Lady and I walked out of chemo and back through the lobby to the vending room to get cheese crackers and peanut M&M's. We walked back through the lobby and into chemo to be greeted with a smile by the Sister as we handed over the goods. Then we went back out of chemo to the lobby. SO—no big deal whatsoever.

We also went repeatedly to a different lobby to tell the Brother to hold his horses because they were running late in pain management and he wanted to just leave. The Lady knew she would be the one the nurse would ask where he had disappeared to and that wasn't fair. The Lady told him so, and by effectively applying the guilt complex, it apparently worked. Then, in-between all that, most of our time was spent making small talk with those around us.

We found Matthew sitting by the front door of the cancer center waiting for a ride home. He sits with a friend who traveled from Corpus Christie to spend time with him. The first thing we find totally out of place is the fact Matthew is wearing a patient bracelet. He's only 28 and a really good-looking kid. With his age and looks of abundant health, he seems out of place here. Curious, the Lady asks what's he doing here. He tells us, today begins his first of four weeks of radiation. We're surprised!

Matthew is married and the father of two little girls who are 3 ½ years and 3 ½ months old. "Gwendolyn and Naomi," he says with pride in his voice. He's been in perfect health for as long as he can remember. He led a very active life by working out four to five times a week. He'd go swimming, camping, bike riding, and he liked spending time at the beach. That all changed one day in December, 2010. On that particular day, he was moving furniture for his mom and thought he'd pulled a muscle in his groin. In the emergency room, he thought they'd get it all taken care of that day and that would be the end of it. They'd fix him up and he'd be on his way! Instead, two days later, he found himself meeting a specialist who told Matthew he either had a tumor or cancer. CT scans revealed he had testicular cancer. Matthew walked back to the waiting room, in a state of shock, to where his father waited for him. When he told his dad he had cancer, he broke down crying. A few months later, in March, he had surgery.

What was his first thought when he found out he had cancer? He thought he was too young to get it; he wasn't old enough for *that*. He was healthy and at an age where you feel invincible! However, his cancer is a genetic one that, according to what his physician told him, commonly strikes males between the ages of 20 to 35.

"I started talking to God (He paused for a moment.) a lot. Asking him, Why ME? Now that I'm working my way through this, it's more, where do I go from here?" Matthew starts getting restless in his chair, exits the area, then returns a short while later. He's not feeling very well. "It must be the treatment," he tells us. The Lady says perhaps a Sprite might make him feel better. Matthew agrees and begins to stand up until the Lady motions for him to sit. We rise and begin our familiar path.

Yours,

Frog

♦　♦　♦　♦　♦　♦　♦　♦

APRIL 22, 2011

Dear Family,

The Sister is an early riser. When it's treatment time, some days it's slow-going getting dressed before she heads straight back to the couch. The only time she hasn't risen early (between 4:00-6:30 a.m.) is after the chemoembolization procedure. During that recovery, she would be awake, but not moving a muscle because of the pain. The Sister struggled through Tuesday, and by late afternoon, she started running a fever. We're suppose to take her to JPS Hospital if it climbs higher than 100.1°F. It climbed past a 100.1°F just as the skies darkened and tornado warning sirens started sounding in the distance. Sirens or not, she just didn't want to go to the hospital.

Back in February, when she was so horribly sick, our gut instinct kept telling us to get her to the hospital, but the Sister refused to go. We didn't know what to do at the time. Squatting down beside the couch, the Lady placed a hand on her arm and got serious. "(Sister's name), if there ever came a time you knew you needed to go to the hospital, you'd tell me, right?" The Sister promised she would. We have to believe that promise still stands on this day. Instead, the Lady and I stood outside watching for tornadoes because the sirens scared the Sister. Outside, the Lady confides it's scarier inside the house not knowing what could be coming toward us. Nothing escapes her notice as we stand in the driveway with her face raised, searching the skies.

Wednesday arrived and the Sister just flat-out didn't get up. At first, the Lady and I circled around by the couch to see if her eyes were open. We have to make a wide berth when we approach because her head is what we see first, and we've accidentally caused her to scream in alarm several times because she didn't hear us coming. On that day, we thought she was sleeping in and were glad for several reasons, but mostly because when she sleeps, she can't be conscious of the nausea or pain. Sometimes I pray she just sleeps; it's easier on my nerves when she sleeps during treatment. Do you think that makes me sound bad? The Sister doesn't feel hot when the Lady touches her so we let her sleep. By 10 a.m., the Lady started getting nervous. By 12:45 p.m., when she still hadn't opened her eyes, we weren't sure what to do. The Lady noticed the fanny pack lying on the floor next to the Sister so she picked it up, unzipping it. Taking the pouch out to see how much drug is left, she notices it's almost empty. The pump was to be disconnected at 3 p.m. The Sister opened her eyes after hearing the zipper being closed on the pack. She mumbled weakly, "I don't know how I'll be able to get to the cancer center." She slowly swings her legs over the side of the couch and sits upright, then doubles over, using her arms as a natural pillow against her lap for her forehead. One, two, three seconds pass before she grabs the spit-up bag and races back to her bathroom.

The Lady decides we're getting the Sister to the cancer center as soon as we can get out the door. By 1:07 p.m. we're in the car. We drive without the radio playing, thinking this would be one of the times it would annoy the Sister. The Lady starts praying in her mind, "Father God, we need a miracle." That's all the further she got in her prayer before she grabbed a tissue and started dabbing her eyes. The Sister asked what was wrong and the Lady told her she couldn't bear to have her wait today to be disconnected. Sometimes it takes *hours* and the thought of having the Sister wait seemed unbearable.

I, too, was in the middle of my own prayer. It went something like this: *Dear GOD! Those drugs are KILLING HER!!! I want that thing OFF her NOW!*

The rest of the trip, I daydreamed about how, one day, the Sister would wake up and her hair and makeup would be perfectly done. It would be as if this past year was just a bad dream and never even happened. She would gather us to her and announce there's no sense in treatments anymore. Sweeping her hands from her shoulders down to her knees, she'd tell us to have a good look, every inch of her was in perfect order inside and out! Praise be! Then I could go home and know the sisters were walking together in the park or going to the movies. They would do what they said they would do—go to Jerusalem together and probably cry over each step they took, all the while wondering if in that exact spot Jesus may have stepped. We would all live really long lives. They'd come and visit us from time to time to make sure I was okay. Then I got scared, wondering if there would come a day when the sister really would say, "Enough! No more treatments!"

This morning at 5:05 a.m., the Lady received a text from Donna. She'll arrive today. Having dipped into her savings account now, Donna recognizes the importance of spending time with her sisters. It's one of those days you won't ever forget, such your wedding date or September 11, 2001. The Lady signs the card, "Baby Girl, I wouldn't have missed one moment of this time with you for anything in this world." We stood at The Cheesecake Factory asking for one slice of cherry for the Sister—her very favorite—even though we both know she won't be eating any of it. If Lou (the nurse we love) were to ever ask, the Lady would be prepared with a date she'll carry through her lifetime and say, "Why, yes! Yes, I *do* recall the exact date. It was April 22. Good Friday. (Pointing to the Sister) Her birthday. She turned 49 that day. It was early that morning that those rotten side effects you warned us about had begun."

Yours,

Frog

P.S. I'm enclosing a gift card for The Cheesecake Factory. The Lady thought it'd be nice if you could go sit at a table (It's really lovely inside.) and enjoy celebrating the Sister's birthday with us by having a piece of cheesecake.

~ Random Blessing: One Sunday, Donna stood waiting in line for sandwiches at a deli, somewhere in New Jersey. Having the strongest feelings about the Sister, it stopped her cold. While running across the parking lot to her car, a shiny dime appeared in her path. She said thank you, kissed it, blessed it, and thought of her sisters in church. Her sisters *were* in church around that time, while Linda was whispering God-sent words into the Sister's ear.

♦ ♦ ♦ ♦ ♦ ♦ ♦ ♦

APRIL 25, 2011

Dear Family,

Ever since the Lady was 5 years old, she's pretended to be "secretary extraordinaire." Excelling in typing and shorthand skills in high school, she carried out her love for paper efficiency into adulthood. She tries to stay on top of thank-you notes amid all else that goes on around here. Last week, she wrote to American Airlines to thank them for allowing us to take pictures in-flight and for making our flight such a special one.

When all the passengers were in their seats, before we had taken off, the male attendant handed us a nice gift bag with a blanket and neck rest inside. When he walked away, the Lady hurried and turned her head toward the window because tears were forming in her eyes. It sounds silly but, for once in a long while, it felt like someone was taking care of *her* this time. The other attendant gave us headphones and told us to enjoy the movie. When the drink/snack cart started making its way down the aisle, we got ready. This was the shot we were wanting! After the picture was taken, the Lady held her debit card in the air and asked for a turkey sandwich. Refusing to take the card, the male attendant said the Vice President wanted her to have it for free.

"Really!?!" she asked.

"Well," the attendant replied, "I'm not sure about that (then he hurried on) but I know if the Vice President *knew* you were onboard, he'd want you to have this."

We couldn't have been more touched by their kindness. The Lady told American Airlines in her thank-you letter, *On that day, the flight attendants were more than employees. They were my family.*

A couple days ago, we got a letter from their corporate office. I really like American Airlines. Read for yourself how nice they are:

(April 19, 2011) . . . Your letter following your trip to visit your daughter was very touching; in fact, I hope you won't mind if I

publish it with my weekly flight attendant update. The crew is truly appreciative of your feedback. Knowing that their simple gestures meant so much to you is what keeps them going with smiles on their faces; it was our pleasure to have you onboard. And in this case, the Vice President WAS aware that (Lady's full name) was flying and I definitely wanted you to enjoy your flight! . . . I'm honored that we could play a small role in your journey.

With warm regards,
Denise Lynn, Vice President, Flight Service

I must tell you this right away because I don't want you to worry! Those rotten side effects the Sister had on the morning of her birthday stopped by noon. The sisters spent all weekend force-feeding her as her little body has dwindled down so much this past week. She, refusing food, says it makes her feel even worse. The refrigerator is stocked with bottles and cartons and flavors of anything she could possibly want. She forces a sip here, a sip there. Pulling Donna aside, the Lady says she's not sure the Sister has gotten 500 calories in her system all week. Donna, no nursing degree needed for this task as she only need be a caring sister, will be the one who knocks on the glass door of Luby's Cafeteria, on Cooper Street, five minutes after closing. She knocks until someone takes pity and opens the door and tells her they're closed. Apologizing, she explains her sister is sick and won't eat, but has agreed to a piece of cornbread and maybe a little corn—if it's not too much trouble. The staff stands listening to her words then, snapping to attention, they make an immediate beeline to the back before returning with hope in their hands as they present the food.

The day after the Sister turned 49, the Lady turned 51. Months out, a mad dash was instigated by the Parents and Donna. Where's the beloved purse? The one with the corndoggy disco ball thingy? It was a limited edition purse and only available for a short time, they were told. Oh no! They wanted the Lady to have it, to give it to her for her birthday, and make this one special! They were unaware that many months back, Renee' and her parents also made this same attempt, but with no luck. A search throughout the United States ensued. Some on-line leads made the family nervous about the authenticity of the purse. Macy's and Coach got involved. Finally, they received word a purse had been located at a Dallas store. Then they were notified there was an error, and that wasn't the right purse. So the search continued until one day, they were filled with joy because a store in Tacoma, Washington, had one left and would ship it shortly.

Now, let me tell you how God works with this family. When the Lady opened the purse on her birthday, she wanted to cry as she picked it up and held it in the air. She was perfectly content to live a lifetime without that purse. She doesn't place much value on worldly things, but (darn!) she liked that purse last July and she likes that purse today. If Donna hadn't bothered to tell the story behind getting this purse into her hands (Tacoma, Washington?), no one would've known that last week the Lady spent a considerable amount of time learning about the American Cancer Society's Relay For Life event. This event has become a big deal in this household. She had told the Sister, only days earlier, that Relay For Life was started by one man, a colorectal surgeon, who ran for 24 hours around a track (83 miles) in support of his patients and to support his local American Cancer Society. One man, Dr. Gordy Klatt, from Tacoma, Washington!

Saturday night, after much discussion of other cases of healing (like the people who get up out of wheelchairs and start walking), the Sister confided to Donna that she wished God would give her a definite sign that she's healing. Just . . . you know, *something*. Sunday morning, she began the long process to get ready for church. She had to sit on the floor and gather strength to brush her hair. The Sister, lacking the energy to stand up and sing, sat during the entire church service. Part way through the singing, the Lady noticed Donna pull a tiny bottled water from her purse and hold to the Sister's lips for a quick sip. The woman behind us made eye contact with the Lady and they smiled at each other over the gesture. Love pours from us toward Donna—a true sister lover.

Don, another "Linda-in-disguise," makes it a point to search the Sister out every Sunday before the service and speak words that mean much. The Lady always thinks, *Boy, I hope that Don guy finds us today!* He's also an inspiration to the Sister and we're not even sure he knows that as he takes her hand in his, "(Sister's name), every morning I pray anointing over your healing. A large group of people here pray for you daily." This Sunday, Easter Sunday, he takes her hand and tells her he's prayed that God would give her a revelation.

"REVELATION!" the Lady says loud enough to startle them.

The Sister smiles because the two of them know the song

Revelation by Third Day is one of the songs she tells us to play over and over when we're in the car. It speaks to her. So when Don used the word *revelation*, a keyword to the Sister, we couldn't help but feel it was God's way of saying pay attention. Listen.

The three sisters make their way through the church foyer after the service; their arms are looped together with the Sister in the middle. The Lady tells them she read Scripture that morning that said something about the cord of two is strong, but the cord of three is unbreakable. "We're the three cords," she tells them. Hearts fill with joy at the thought.

That night by the flickering light of the TV, Donna started gathering her laptop and other belongings from off the living room floor to begin packing. She stopped and looked at the Sister on the couch and tears came. "I don't want to leave you, (Sister's name). I don't want to leave you. My heart is here with you."

Yours,

Frog

♦ ♦ ♦ ♦ ♦ ♦ ♦ ♦

APRIL 27, 2011

Dear Family,

This happened a long time ago during the time the Sister and Brother were going through radiation. One day, the Lady sat biding her time in the waiting room when Tera (the radiation receptionist at that time) approached. She'd found something that weekend while shopping with her aunt at a garage sale, two little matching frog ornaments. When she saw the pair she thought of us and wanted the Lady to have them. Her aunt, as Tera would tell, is a woman filled with the spirit of the Lord and for years *her* source for spiritual guidance. Telling her aunt about me, she asked if a frog could be used for God's purpose. Brenda told her she thinks God can use anything you believe in and whatever it takes to send His love and healing power to those who ask and believe. When Tera walked away, the Lady looked down at the little frogs in her hand. They made her smile. Noticing some of their tiny toes were broken off and missing, it hadn't made them any less loved. I think it's the same with people. God sees the ones who are broken and the ones who have been missing and He loves them just the same.

<u>Angie's Story</u>:
This is how Angie was described to me. Angie was an amazing woman in her early 50s. She was a mother of two, grandmother of two, a devout Christian, a member of Sugar Hill Baptist Church, and a faculty member at North Gwinnett High School. Angie kept a tiny, little tree on her desk at work and would decorate it throughout the year according to seasons or holidays. Bringing joy to others, loved by many, she was a strong woman, a real fighter. Her fight began when she was diagnosed with uterine cancer. Angie never gave up. She began chemo treatments and almost never missed a day of work because of it. The school kept a cot in the back area of the office for her in case she ever needed to lie down. She had such incredible

determination to beat this thing. The school rallied behind her and participated in the American Cancer Society's Relay For Life (RFL) event that year.

They had 25 team members and raised $6,230. They were in it for Angie. Angie passed away in June of 2006 and wouldn't live to see the school rally behind her memory the following year at RFL. She couldn't possibly know that five years later, the school would be one of the top high schools in the nation to support RFL. Last year, they raised $50,000, and this year, with over 200 team members, they are rallying for $70,000. Incredible as it sounds, with over 20 countries participating in RFL, Gwinnett County, Georgia, holds the largest one-night event in the WORLD raising over $2 million last year, $1 million coming from their schools alone. Some, such as Carol, would never forget Angie's words stressing the importance of continuing RFL. *It won't help me but it will help someone else.*

On weekdays, you'll find Carol in her office at North Gwinnett High. On a table in her office sits Angie's tree. It's decorated for Easter. When Angie passed away, the school set up a scholarship in her memory. Angie was always so proud of Carol's daughter, Katie. Katie dreamed of becoming a registered nurse and someday working with pediatric cancer patients. A few years later, Katie graduated from NGHS and Angie's scholarship helped pay for her nursing school.

Carol still misses Angie. This year she'll participate in her sixth 24-hour RFL event. It will be her fifth since Angie's passing. RFL is actually a year-long event at the school with various events held to raise money throughout the year. The grand finale, the actual relay, will be held at the Gwinnett County Fair Grounds on May 6.

Being a lifelong friend of this family and best friend to Donna in high school (NGHS), Carol picked up the phone one night and called the Lady. Each year Carol chooses someone to represent. This year, she (and she'll say, *I'm one of MANY!*) will be raising money and walking in honor of the Sister. "I want to give her another birthday." When the call ends, the Lady becomes emotional as she relays this news to the Sister. Tears come to their eyes and they're touched by such thoughtfulness. Well, truthfully, I cried too! Because the Sister's cancer is a rare one, they don't often hear of research toward hers. During one of our walks together, long ago in the park, the Sister voiced her concern about what if no one was trying to find a cure for her type since so few have it. We started to leave the room when a quiet voice asked, "Do you think it'll (the money) go toward my cancer, too?" The Lady smiles and tells her, "Yes, honey. I'm sure it goes toward all of them."

This is a big deal, people representing the Sister in the world's largest RFL event of the year. The Lady wishes either one of us could attend, but we've never, EVER been separated since the Lady found me—well, except for the one Sunday she left me in her purse, in the car, instead of taking me into church. She fretted all during the service because she couldn't remember if she locked the car and was worried sick someone would steal me. How would she explain that to you? I was fine, but she vowed she'd never leave me again and she hasn't.

"Heeey!" I told the Lady, "Since we can't attend, maybe we should send one of the missing-toes-twins to Carol. He could stand in for us!"

Great idea!! A frog twin left the very next morning. Hello Suwanee, Georgia!

Yours,

Frog

♦ ♦ ♦ ♦ ♦ ♦ ♦ ♦

APRIL 30, 2011

Dear Family,

One night, last November, the Lady received an e-mail from her close friend, Victoria, in Illinois. It was one of those e-mails that are forwarded and circulated around the Internet. When Victoria read it, she said it reminded her of us. The Lady has received the same e-mail several times since from others claiming the same thing. After reading the story Victoria sent, the Lady was surprised. Of course it wasn't written about *us,* but there are vague similarities. So, even though this isn't about US, it means, well, we can only conclude, there is a younger/cuter version of "sorta the two of us" somewhere out there in this world! If this story is true, then what a coincidnce! We love it. Here's the story:

I was told a story about a lady in the hospital who was near death when an area Chaplain came to visit her. This Chaplain was a very young female with long blond hair. She listened to the lady who was ill and left her a small gift for comfort. It was a tiny ceramic frog. The next day, one of the people from the lady's church came to visit. The lady told her friend about the beautiful young Chaplain who had come to visit her. The friend was so impressed with the way the lady had improved she felt the need to talk to the young Chaplain. In her search to find the young woman, she was repeatedly reassured that the chaplains are never very young and that there was never a woman that fit the description given. Upon returning to the lady in the hospital, a visiting nurse entered the room and noticed the ceramic frog. The nurse made the comment, "I see you have a guardian angel with you." As she held the little frog, we asked why she made the comment and we were informed that the frog stood for: (F) Forever (R) Rely (O) On (G) God. (Author Unknown)

The Lady said she sees my letters to you in a totally different light after reading that e-mail. She'd never thought of a frog standing for that but maybe Tera's aunt was right—God can use whatever means

He chooses to get His word out. You know, you could've chosen any number of things to put on our mailbox—a gnome, a snail, whatever, and it just wouldn't have worked. With me being a frog, I was exactly the right thing to tell this story. I'm telling you, God doesn't make mistakes.

I'll do a quick update on everyone right now:

The Dad continues to have blood clots in his legs. He takes Coumadin every night. His legs swell up with a good day/bad day guess from one day to the next. His physician says the blood clots will probably never go away. His heavenly physician says nothing is impossible and nothing is too big. The first Monday of every month he sits for the Zometa IV infusion to help build up his bones. The M-Spike (marker test for cancer) still registers zero!

The Mom, as always, continues to be caregiver to the Dad—his helpmate for life. On any chance that presents itself, she witnesses to those who cross her path and tells others of the healings within her family. One Sunday, the pastor of her church asked her to share her testimony on how God has sustained her family. As she scurries around in her busy life, any casual observer is likely to catch her leaving little faith-based pamphlets here and there for others to find (and hopefully read) after she leaves. Her faith is strong.

The Brother briefly returned here then left again to spend more time with his daughter. She miscarried his first grandchild and he's helping her cope with the loss. His heart isn't here with us. The sisters tell him they want him to be happy, wherever that is.

Donna returned to New Jersey. She sent a text: *Got my pillow out of the suitcase and it smelled like (Sister's name) house. Made me wanna cry. I never have more fun, laugh more, relax more, or enjoy anyone's company more than when I am with you two. You are precious to me!* Three cords, remember?

The Sister took five days to eat her piece of birthday cheesecake before snapping out of her bout with anorexia. She's eaten like a horse for four days now. We're all relieved as chemo starts again on Monday. I heard the sisters talking about more Bible questions and interesting facts they are discovering. One night, they were reading and talking about angels (again) when the oldest nephew interrupted to ask why Enoch got to go straight to heaven without dying. That question came out of the clear blue because Enoch hadn't even been brought up. The Sister said she'd look it up, but *first* she was going to finish what she was reading about angels. Looking down to where her finger rested on a page in the Bible was the very verse about Enoch. Her finger randomly resting on it! Stuff like that happens here constantly.

Another time, the Sister said, when they go to heaven, Jesus is going to give each person a white rock with their new name on it, a secret name no one else knows but Him. The Lady asked her if she'd tell her her secret name and they started laughing because the Lady said if she *didn't* tell—there's a chance she would sneak into the Sister's house when she's not home and rummage through her drawers looking for the rock. It was funny. What I thought was really sweet is her name now. We found out the Sister's name means *Light As The Day*. The Mom and Dad named her appropriately. She is light.

The Lady says she had the best, best birthday this year. She told everyone including the Fed Ex driver, a complete stranger, who was only trying to deliver a package. With Friday being the Sister's birthday, Saturday *her* birthday, and Sunday being Easter, it will be hard to beat those three consecutive days of celebration. Every day she gets up and tells me to have a look at the world, really look at it, because it's beautiful. Never forget to give thanks and pay attention during the day. Be on the lookout for God signs in our lives. Not just BIG signs, but the small ones too, that reassure us He's constantly listening to us and aware of our every need. He'll show you in some way if you'll just pay attention. For instance, remember the time I was holed up all those days because of the Lady's sinus infection? She was hacking and coughing hard as she lay in bed. One afternoon, she reached for her phone and texted the younger nephew asking, if he happened to get out, could he bring her some lemon cough drops. When she tossed the phone back down, it dawned on her she didn't mean *lemon* cough drops. She doesn't care so much for those and meant to say honey-flavored, but figured she'd endure lemon this time because she felt too miserable bothering to retext. Later, the nephew tapped on the door, sticking only his arm in for fear he'd catch a germ, and tossed a package onto the dresser. "Sorry, this is all I saw," he said, then quickly shut the door. The Lady got up to grab the bag and smiled. Yep, you got it, honey-flavored. Honestly!

Did you realize on Monday, one year ago, I came home with the Lady? On Tuesday, one year ago, I wrote you my first letter home. Nuts! Huh? I had no idea what the past year would hold. I thought I'd write to you for a couple months, then one morning you'd wake up and SURPRISE, I'd be back in my spot on the mailbox. I laugh now as I type this. Who could have known? With everyone getting well around us, the Lady decided we'd better have my right eye looked at by a professional, you know, just as a precaution. She's always been half afraid I'd lose it. This morning we went to Matlock Oaks Animal Clinic and Dr. Garrett thinks I'm in pretty good shape. The Lady will continue to monitor my right eye, but it shouldn't fall out anytime soon.

Yours,

Frog

♦   ♦   ♦   ♦   ♦   ♦   ♦   ♦

MAY 4, 2011

Dear Family,

"You know what I was thinking about? See if you remember this." The Lady looked up from her spot on the floor where she was reading, giving the Sister her full attention. "Remember when we were really young they had a contest at church for the kids? At Emma Baptist? And you picked the smallest doll contest?"

"Oh my gosh! I *do* remember that! How do you? It was so long ago."

It's chemo week and the pump is dispensing. While lying on her back, the Sister continues her story as if she's speaking to the ceiling.

"I saw you rummaging all through the toy box trying to find a really small doll. When I saw how badly you tried to find one so you could win a prize, I made you one (turning her head toward us), remember that?"

"Yeah, I totally remember that now, but I'd completely forgotten about it. What was it made out of? A little piece of tissue?"

"No, I think it was a piece of a white sheet or t-shirt. I got a small black bead for the head and used a string to tie the cloth around it."

"Yeah, that's *right*. It looked like a little bitty ghost doll."

"And it was so small we didn't want it to get ruined so we put it in a little box to carry it to church."

"A box that held jewelry. It had cotton lining the bottom." (What happened to that doll? Did she just chuck it like it had no importance? The thought makes her sick so she starts to cry at her carelessness. She would have kept it forever had she known . . .)

"And I got a pen and marked the face with eyes and stuff. I wasn't sure they'd accept it as a real doll, but I think you won!"

The Lady, thinking to herself, *and I bet I never even thanked her for doing that because I was so bent on getting a prize.*

By late Tuesday afternoon, the Sister was lying in her bathroom, cheek pressed against the cold tile, and body wrapped in blankets to combate her chills. The Lady and Sister decided it may do more damage to pile on more blankets since she was warm to the touch. She remained on the floor throughout the night. The following morning, she decided she was going to just lay on the couch until it was time to have the pump disconnected. It was Wednesday morning. The clock read 8:56 a.m., and the Sister was sick to her stomach. In the midst of the Lady checking on her, straightening up the house, and starting laundry, our thoughts drifted to JPS Hospital first floor radiology.

If we were there this moment, we'd find our friend Kim in the waiting area. She's two hours away from undergoing chemoembolization to her liver. Last week, when the Lady spoke to her on the phone, Kim confided she told her doctor not to give up on her just yet. According to her, five percent with her type cancer beat it. Someone has to be in that five percent and it might as well be her! After she left the doctor's office, she picked out future birthday and graduation cards for her three children and made a mental list of what she'd want each child to have for future birthday gifts. This brought her comfort. She was taking care of something she'd wanted to do for a while now. Kim doesn't see her actions as a lack of faith in her healing. Her faith is strong. She says we *all* have to die someday and she wants to be ready. She went to Build-A-Bear Workshop and selected a stuffed frog for her oldest son. For the two younger ones, she spent time making them a talking teddy bear. She recorded words her children could play back and listen to when she was no longer around. These words are special words she's told them all their lives. The Lady smiled when Kim repeated them to her because they were spoken with such love flowing from her voice:

"I love you BIG as the WORLD, TALL as the SKY, to the MOON and BACK, from the TIPS of your TOES, and EVERYTHING inbetween . . . "

Yours,

Frog

❖ ❖ ❖ ❖ ❖ ❖ ❖ ❖

DianaRae   189

MAY 14, 2011

Dear Family,

Monday started chemo week again and I was not looking forward to it. The last Monday we were at the cancer center, the Lady and I had an unsavory experience. Way back when the Dad was first diagnosed with cancer, Donna called and told the Lady to beware. A lot of sickness comes from the devil and being among all that sickness could be a threat to their spiritual well-being. Well, I heard the Lady say/snort into the phone, "Pfffffhhh! No . . . It's not like that here!" At that point, we'd been hanging around lots of sick people for months and nothing weird had happened. That all changed that one Monday.

We were sitting there minding our own business while eavesdropping on the conversation of two women who sat a chair away from us. Occasionally, a couple words would float our way until it became apparent they were talking about the Bible. It wasn't long before the four of us were chatting. The Lady, I'm telling you, has no control over this. She went into this big speech about their family and what God had done (hardly pausing for breath) then ended by wiping a tear from her eye.

One woman left to place a phone call while the other woman moved on to another subject. (If by chance you have the soundtrack from the movie Jaws—I suggest you begin playing it while reading what happened next.) She started talking about spiritual warfare and occult occurrences she'd encountered in the past. The more she talked, the more I started wondering exactly which "side of the war" she was on! She continued by discussing this priestess she knew who was powerful. She went on and on, until it got to the part when she said the priestess's eyes changed colors when she talked. I got creeped out and kept expecting the shades on the windows to start rolling up and down in quick succession all on their own! The Lady interrupted and said she didn't want to hear another word. We left right away. It was so creepy!

I've already told you about last Tuesday night and how the Sister slept with her cheek pressed against the bathroom floor tile. That night, the Lady went to lie down and began to pray when the words *"The blood of Jesus is flowing through her veins,"* entered her mind. The words came through strong, with such a powerful message because the blood of Jesus is pure and a giver of life. Each time she repeated the words, she became more humbled and sure God's hand was on the Sister right that moment as she lay sick on the floor with her chemo pump dispensing. He was aware of her every need and cleansing her blood and giving her life.

That Wednesday, we entered the cancer center to have the pump disconnected, but the Sister's blood pressure was too low. They ran something through her port in an attempt to raise it; otherwise, she'd have to be hospitalized. Listen to this, when we got home, the Sister immediately went to the couch and sat down. The Lady stood in the kitchen humming a song, while eating an individual serving size pineapple cup over the sink, when we heard a noise.

"What was that?" the Sister asked.

The Lady walked to the living room and said, "Maybe something hit the door."

"No," the Sister said, *"I thought it came from where you were."*

The Lady started back toward the kitchen when she saw a candle from a wall sconce lying on the floor. She picked it up and told us it was *this* candle; it just jumped right off the wall! We all laughed as the Lady put it back in place then sat on the floor across from us. The Sister asked what if that was the Holy Spirit. Immediately, the Lady drew in a sharp breath after remembering what she was humming the exact moment the candle fell. She told us she has a new song stuck in her head called *Blessings* by Laura Story. She doesn't know many of the words yet except for a phrase that says something like, *What if your healing comes from God?* Those were the words she was humming!

Thursday, I went with the Lady to Dr. Glover's office and guess what happened for the third time while we were waiting in our room? You guessed it! A dove flew down and walked around in front of the window. That reminded us of the Dad again.

Saturday's text from the Dad: *Flowers just arrived, pretty 2lips. Went out 4 breakfast (The Skillet in Ballentyne), Phil Mickelson sat next to us. That's all the excitement your Mom can handle this week. Lv dad*

Who's Phil? we text back.

The Dad replies: *He's one of the five best golfers in the world. Wanted to ask him about his wife, she's been battling cancer for some time now, but didn't want to bother him.*

Sunday was Mother's Day. Did you get my card? We went to church and Don came to where we were sitting and was speaking to the Sister when he said, "... *the blood of Jesus* ... " and the Lady whipped her face to the Sister and said, "the BLOOD of JE-sus!" The Sister knows the Lady's been saying those words every day for her and we weren't sure if this was another God sign or if Linda (who's also claiming these words) had told Don earlier.

After church, we went to brunch at Mimi's Cafe with the Lady's son's girlfriend, Sarah, and her Aunt Marsha. When we got home, the Sister wanted to know if Linda had already spoken with Don before he saw us. She *had* to know. Was it or was it not a God sign? Checking with Linda, she confirmed she'd told no one so it must be a God sign!

Okay, this letter turned out way too long, but I haven't written home in a while.

Yours,

Frog

♦ ♦ ♦ ♦ ♦ ♦ ♦ ♦

MAY 20, 2011

Dear Family,

The answer to the question, *Should I continue treatment or not?*, was perhaps known all along within the deep recesses of the Sister's mind. Lying wait, precariously balanced, and ready to tilt one way (the familiar way) or veer startlingly off the other way (into the unknown). Anything could uneven the scales at a moment's notice. If the Sister happened to be reading a particularly interesting book or Scripture, the scales might tilt toward treatment. Brushing out her wig could tilt the scales the opposite way. On Sundays, the scales would tilt wildly back in the other direction and gain some leverage. No longer comfortable with the way her pants fit would result in leverage from Sundays being lost. Cherry cheesecake placed in front of her, when she was able to eat, would send the scales happily back. Basically, it comes down to her mood. If she's content, she'll continue on. If she's miserable, she wants to stop.

One morning last week, as the Lady and I sat at the computer, the Sister walked in and announced she wasn't so sure she'd continue treatment any longer. The chemo was ruining her body; plus, she thought her other tumor might be growing because something inside just didn't feel right. The Lady and I remained silent, lips zipped, holding our breath. Truthfully, neither of us had given the other tumor any thought at all lately, considering it dead or gone—body healed. She continued, "I'm just going to wait for God to give me a sign about what to do. I've already prayed about that." (We can breathe again.) It's occurred to all of us, the Sister included, that the symptoms from which she suffers aren't from the cancer itself. The culprit is chemo. Remove all the contaminates from her bloodstream and odds are, odds are . . . I don't know *what* the odds are. Perhaps she'd become a normal-functioning person with the blood of Jesus flowing through her veins. From that day on, the Sister's referred to her cancer in past tense. *"When I HAD cancer . . . "*

DianaRae   193

Once it became apparent we were headed back for another round of treatment on Monday, I went over my newly formulated "plan of entry" with the sisters. Having no desire whatsoever for another repeat waiting room experience such as the last creepy one, I concocted the following suggestion: We should all adorn hastily constructed (yet in totally good taste) necklaces made out of bulbs of garlic—surely available in the produce section at Albertsons. Then (I especially liked this part), while humming to the tune of *Holy Is The Lord* by Chris Tomlin, the Lady would lead our entourage into the cancer center while waving back and forth an 8 x 12 inch cross in her outstretched arm, sweeping a safe passage to our seating. Well! That idea got vetoed immediately as the sisters mutually agreed they'd not put a vegetable or piece of metal in charge of our safety! Their God is mighty, remember? Oh yeah, what was I thinking?

By the way, again we heard that *Blessings* song I told you about in my last letter. The Lady was humming the right words for the "eating-pineapple-at-the-kitchen-sink-moment" BUT they weren't the actual right words to the song.

Yours,

Frog

♦ ♦ ♦ ♦ ♦ ♦ ♦ ♦

MAY 31, 2011

Dear Family,

You would think I'd have a plausible reason for the 11-day lapse between letters and the least I could do is send a picture. No excuse here. Sorry. Busted. I got sidetracked reading a 500-page book about the former First Lady, Laura Bush. It was fiction, which means I read certain pieces that literally stunned me until I remembered it was all pretend dialog, etc. Nevertheless, I read it during all my free time and couldn't quite put it down until the last page was turned. So, that's where I've been, pretty much sitting over here with my nose stuck in a book!

It made me so sad to hear the Sister talking one afternoon last week. She was talking about her life and the struggles she's gone through because she's so shy. The Sister speaks softly with no trace of animosity in her tone. No hooping, hollering, or fist pounding on the table. Her face doesn't even squinch up the way I've seen others when relaying sorrowful tales about themselves. This passive acceptance she has toward the stories—these stories, her stories—make them all the more drastic to me as they unfold. I'll share a couple of these with you because the subject is rarely discussed. You know how a small child is defenseless against adults? Their well-being is at the mercy of those far larger. Do you know there are people in the world who are defenseless adults because they're incredibly shy? It never dawned on me that this could happen. Have you ever thought about that?

We, I say *we* since it affects us all, made it past the last treatment only to face the next round starting today—a day late due to the Memorial Day holiday. Every other week comes sooner for a cancer patient than, say, every other week by a well person's calendar. A week-and-a-half recovery time is not nearly enough. We hope this treatment starts without a hitch compared to the last time when the Sister's blood pressure (80/50) was too low to even begin treatment without first draining something through her port. That Tuesday night (always

Tuesday nights), she lay on her bathroom floor uncovered because of fever-induced chills, even though she'd prefer to be wrapped in a cocoon of blankets. The thermometer registers over 102°F. Moments earlier, a text was sent to Donna. Combating fevers with over-the-counter drugs are tricky if the patient has liver problems. Should a double dose be given at the start, giving it a little "punch" in the beginning? Fevers cause dehydration, and dehydration causes fevers. The Lady squats down next to the Sister while shaking a single pill from a bottle of ibuprofen. Ziploc bags of ice cubes, wrapped in a t-shirt, are placed on her forehead. A bottle of Gatorade is placed next to the Sister with instructions to start drinking and keep drinking until it's gone. Two prayers are issued, and within 45 minutes, no temperature is registered. In fact, it's slightly below normal.

Looking back (third grade), the Sister sits at a desk in her classroom. Her pencil, positioned in her left hand, moves slowly across the paper from left to right. Her right arm, resting on the desk, curves around her notebook paper as if she were guarding the words she writes. Her head is bent down as she quietly works on the assignment. With no warning, a hand from behind grabs a fistful of hair, yanking her head back. Words are crossly directed at her to keep her head up! Tears pool in the Sister's eyes. Mortified, she looks at no one, telling no one this story until now.

The best I can say health-wise, during the past week-and-a-half recovery time, is new baby hair is growing. We scan the Sister's head noting she didn't lose all of her hair, but it's very thin. The new hair, thickest above her forehead, is about two inches long. The Lady, to be funny, says if we flat iron it we might get it to three inches. It's close to her natural hair color but nothing like its former texture; it appears in really small, tight waves. Other than that, daily, the Sister wakes exhausted partly due to waking during the night with loud ringing in her ears and tingling in her fingers and toes. One morning, she came out of her restroom and needed to be led to the couch. Her vision was off; she felt cross-eyed. Once she was seated, she asked the Lady to have a look at her eyes. Did they look cross-eyed to her? No, no they didn't, but as the Lady got up to leave, she turned her head and crossed her own eyes to see for herself what the Sister was feeling at that moment.

The area between her ribcage feels bloated, as if she'd finished a Thanksgiving feast, yet her stomach is empty. It makes her miserably uncomfortable as she waits for whatever is bloating inside her to get to the point it explodes! It certainly feels like that's a real possibility and could happen.

The Sister's losing weight so the Lady buys her a pair of white slacks for church. Back in the day, she wore a size 5/6. Guessing, we buy a size 4. Exchanging them for a size 2, she slips them on and we realize a size 1 or 0 would've fit better. We don't bother returning the size 2, figuring she'll need them when she starts gaining weight.

The Sister was a young mom living in Joliet, Illinois, 30 years ago. One day after work, she decided to stop and get her hair cut before going home. Picking a random, small salon near her neighborhood, she entered the empty salon with only one stylist on duty—the owner. The Sister, following the woman to the sink and reclining to have her hair washed, was unaware she would endure anything more than the usual beauty salon procedure. The stylist proceeded from the get-go to man-handle her. She washed her hair with extreme roughness then, afterward, hatefully ripped the comb through the Sister's hair. She angrily tapped her chin to the left or right to move the Sister's head, pulling hard on her hair as she cut it. The Sister sat paralyzed in the chair. She spoke not a word, didn't cry out, or give any indication anything was amiss at all. Frozen, she sat and endured undeserved abuse because she didn't speak out—*couldn't* speak out—couldn't *speak*. Sure, she wanted to say something—confront the stylist who was a complete stranger, but she was gripped with fear. There'd be no confrontation. There could never *be* because the words, perfectly formulated in her mind, could never be masterly delivered. No amount of mistreatment could trigger her into action. When the stylist finished, the Sister rose from the chair, quietly paid for the cut, then drove home and burst into tears at what she'd gone through.

"What was her name? Do you remember?" the Lady asked of the Sister.

For what purpose does she ask this? What's she going to do at *this* late date? Call this unknown woman and play the 20 questions game? Why'd she do it? How could she have *done* that? How *could* she? Why the Sister? Why *her*? What'd she ever do to *you*? The Sister couldn't remember the woman's name, if she had ever known.

Health-wise, the worst I can say isn't even on that list of side effects, the rotten ones, for this new drug. I was thinking the chemo drug entered the system, filtered through the liver, went this-a-way and that-a-way, then mysteriously vanished into the bloodstream like, ideally, the old drug seemed to do. The reality of this new drug is, eventually it exits the body in a gel-type form that comes out feeling like molten hot lava capable of burning the skin. A gel that, according to the Sister, feels like acid the moment it touches the skin. You'd think after it wound its way all through the body it'd be a mere shell of its former potency. Not so. It leaves the body while giving the impression it's only just begun its journey.

It wasn't long after her 90-day probationary period at the law firm, the attorney entered the Sister's office and handed her a form to fill out for medical insurance. She filled it out within days and placed it on a secretary's desk. A long while would pass until the attorney approached the Sister to question her, noticing she still wasn't showing up on their insurance program. She explained she'd filled out the paperwork a long time ago. The Sister was an efficient employee, but she was also shy. She minded her own business and didn't get involved in office politics between others that, according to her, sometimes ended in raised voices and slammed doors. Perhaps it was her unwillingness to gossip, or take sides, or maybe it was something as simple as her lack of flashy clothes, but someone wasn't willing to complete her medical insurance enrollment. She couldn't muster the thought of confronting the secretary or the attorney on her behalf.

Years would pass when one day, quite suddenly, the attorney passed away and the Sister was grieved over this (still is). Another equally liked attorney stepped up to take over the practice. The offices were moved, people were let go, and insurance benefits (the ones she never had) were dropped in an attempt to keep the firm operating. When everything settled down, the Sister was grateful she still had her job. She loved her job and the people in the office. "If only I'd had insurance all those years," she told us, "I would've gone to the doctor for my yearly exams. I *know* I would have. Then maybe (*Maybe* comes out as a half-sob/half-word.) they would've caught my tumor when it was just stage one."

The Lady partially rises and, walking on her knees across the space that separates them, puts her arms around the Sister. Drawing her close, she buries her face in the Sister's shoulder and starts to weep great sobs as the Sister pats her back and whispers, "I know. I know life's not always fair."

Sometimes I get carried away when I write home. I *know* this. It'll cross my mind and I'll question myself. Why put forth such an effort repeating the tales of this family's todays and yesterdays? I mean, why bother? Truthfully, I kid myself when I feign ignorance that I don't have the answer. I know *exactly* why. I want you to know her for always.

Yours,

Frog

P. S. Remember back when the Sister had the 10 best healthy days since I've been here? I never told you, but during all the running around to the movies and everywhere else we went during those great days, one day was especially nice. We had breakfast at Ol' South Pancake House, in Ft. Worth. Then we went on the train ride through Trinity River Park. The sisters want you to experience the same wonderful morning we did. Enclosed is a gift card for breakfast at Ol' South Pancake along with tickets for the train ride. You'll love it! Finally, since I've been gone over a year now, I need to know if you want me to keep writing home or stop now. If you want me to keep writing home and stay here a while longer with this family, please tie the enclosed pink ribbon on our mailbox flag and leave it on for about a week. We'll drive by and check.

◆ ◆ ◆ ◆ ◆ ◆ ◆ ◆

JUNE 3, 2011

Dear Family,

The Sister's appointment to start chemo on Tuesday was scheduled for 12:30 p.m. Because Monday was Memorial Day, the center was closed. They were running very behind by almost three hours. Well, technically, 30 minutes of that was due to an entirely different reason.

The three of us were sitting in the first couple of chairs as you enter the first waiting room on the chemo side. It wasn't too long before the Lady turned toward the Sister and said, "You smell that?" (Both sisters start exaggerated inhaling.)

"I smell . . . something," the Sister said.

"Smells like natural gas. (Nostrils inflate with more inhaling.) If we smell it long enough it'll put us to sleep and, eventually, we'll die."

Surveying the room, the Sister starts pointing out people who are yawning, had chins resting on their palms, and various others who were flat out slumped over asleep. We start laughing.

"See? Everyone's already falling asleep!" the Lady said in a joking tone, until she spied a woman sitting across the aisle, five chairs down, with her shirt drawn up over her nose. They make eye contact. "You smell it too?" the Lady asked. The woman nodded her head up and down.

The registration office was closed for lunch and the lights were off so the Lady stood and walked around the corner. Recognizing the housekeeping lady, we approached.

"Some of us out here smell something. It kinda smells like natural gas," the Lady told her.

We returned and sat down next to the Sister. Lou (the nurse) appeared in the entryway behind us and, speaking to someone else, we overheard someone say, "Yeah, I smell something real strong over in this area." Moments later Dr. Choufani appeared, waved at us, then joined in trying to (I can only guess) determine if there was cause for concern. Shortly after, an office manager appeared to address our waiting room, "We are evacuating the building. The fire department has been called. Please calmly leave the building."

Everyone, and I mean ev-er-y-one, begins making their way to the nearest exit doors located on all sides of the building. Patients, caregivers, medical and office personnel alike, congregate outside. It's hot outside so the Lady leads the Sister over to a tree and tells her to have a seat on the concrete curb. Within minutes, we hear sirens approaching from the distance—closer, closer, closer until the police and fire department pull up.

After inspecting the building, they give an "All Clear" so patients, caregivers, medical and office staff begin re-entering the building. The Lady and I get separated from the Sister in the rush of bodies and fall behind. A male employee, holding the door open for everyone, let us know as we walked past that nothing was found—no cause for alarm. However, just before we crossed the threshold, a woman standing by the outside brick column told the man holding the door, "Why, I even smelled it earlier when I was standing right here— outside!" The Lady overheard this and her face becomes stricken. When we get back inside the waiting room, we're delighted the Sister picked out new, even better seats this time so we can see the TV. The wait begins again. About another hour and a half into the wait, I see the Lady tap the Sister and overhear her story:

"This morning I was out of my cucumber-melon body mist spray so I threw the bottle in the trash and grabbed this new one I'd bought. (She pulls a small gingery-smelling bottle from her purse and quickly shows the Sister before sliding it back out of view.) When we were walking back into the building, I heard a woman say she smelled the natural gas outside earlier where she was standing by the brick column. (Leaning in close to the Sister, she now speaks in a barely audible whisper.) I sprayed that body mist on me before I entered the building. (Reenactment in her mind: Approaching front door, almost to brick column, takes body mist out of purse, throws chin in the air, squirt, squirt, entered building, sat down, 1-2-3 . . . 20, *You smell that?*) I think maybe my perfume was that natural gas smell . . . "

The Sister looked at her and started giggling then says, "Surely it wasn't the spray!"

"I can't be, like, *arrested* or anything for that, can I?" the Lady asked.

Granted, it wasn't exactly the same as evacuating a McDonald's.

Yours,

Frog

~ Random Blessing: We saw your act of kindness (in the only way you had to communicate with me). You chose NOT to tie the pink ribbon on our mailbox flag. Instead, you lovingly tied the ribbon around the entire mailbox! When we told the Sister about it on Wednesday, even though she wasn't feeling well, she insisted we drive by so she could see it too. As we drove away, she said it made her feel like crying. That was so sweet.

◆　◆　◆　◆　◆　◆　◆　◆

Dear Family,

<u>Chemo Week Symptom Checklist:</u>
Nausea—√
Vomiting—√
Fatigue—√
Fever—√
Loss of appetite—√
Spirits down—√
Weight loss—√
Bloating between ribs—√
Liver pain—√
Low blood pressure—√
Chemo brain—√*
* *Chemo brain* is our term for memory loss, foggy head, confusion, not-all-together-right-in-your-mind feeling.

With chemo week behind us, the Sister's fifth treatment on the new drug since April, the Lady asked if records show what the game plan is for this new drug. A nurse looks over the Sister's chart. She tells us the doctor wants to continue this drug every other week for six months, but this will probably be the last treatment before tests are run to see if it's working. We think this would be an excellent time for scans and, until that happens, daydream of prayers answered and scans revealing a miracle—proof for all to see she's cancer-free! However, after visiting Dr. Choufani yesterday, he told us scans will be done after three more treatments (six more weeks). So, here we go . . .

Last week, the Sister asked the Lady if she had a bucket list. Years ago, the Lady made just such a list, but she barely remembered what was on it. One thing for sure, she wanted to be with their Grandmother during her final moments on earth—hold her hand.

"What about you?" the Lady asked.

The Sister's Bucket List so far:
~ Create a small butterfly sanctuary
~ Pet and maybe ride a horse again
~ Ride a moped
~ See the ocean once again
~ Go to Disneyland once again
~ Swim in a pool once again

The Sister's done some recent research on how to lure butterflies to the house. Well, not just *any* butterfly. She wants to attract Monarchs, Black Swallowtail, and the Painted and American Ladies varieties. You need a host plant for the butterfly to lay eggs (they're picky) and an adult food plant to host the caterpillars until they transform. The Ladies varieties use thistle for both their host and food plant, while the Swallowtail uses certain herb plants as a host and thistle as their food.

Knowing the Sister doesn't have the energy right now to make this happen, and the "butterfly business" isn't a year-round happening, the Lady and I checked all the local garden centers for thistle. No one had thistle. We *needed* thistle! As we were driving home that day, the Lady happened to notice thistle growing wild on the side of the road! Setting her alarm for early the next morning, we sneaked out of the house, loaded a bucket, gloves, and a shovel into her trunk, and drove away. Locating the spot at the side of the road, she pulled over, walked down into the ditch, and started repeatedly stabbing the ground with the shovel. It made me a nervous wreck. We might look suspicious (as in trying to bury evidence of some sort) and someone (possibly the ditch owners) might pull up and meanly yell, "Hey you! What's going on down there?" More stabbing and more stabbing went on, but no matter how hard the Lady tried, it was like trying to break concrete. The ground was too hard! We drove back home, empty-handed, to research what else we could try. Milkweed!

Arriving at Mansfield Nursery, the clerk lead us to the milkweed and also suggested rue. Both are host plants for the type of butterfly the Sister wants. Filled with gladness at another successful mission, the Lady confides to Cynthia, the clerk, "I'm so happy I feel like crying!" Wanting to surprise the Sister, we rush home to assemble the milkweed, rue, parsley, and dill in the privacy of the garage. However, while unloading our supplies, the Lady hit her head hard on the partially closed garage door. While pressing on the crown of her head, then looking at her fingers for any trace of blood (this called for a blood injury; it hurt *that* bad so blood should certainly be involved), the Sister came out to investigate the racket. Looking over the plants, she told us this was going to be better than she imagined. Although we kept checking all throughout the days since, we haven't had any visitors to our sanctuary except a persistent bee and a grasshopper the Lady flicked off the dill. The Lady said if we didn't get any action soon, we might have to invest in a net and stage the whole thing just to make the Sister happy. Anyway, Butterfly Sanctuary—√!

Yours,

Frog

♦ ♦ ♦ ♦ ♦ ♦ ♦ ♦

JUNE 18, 2011

Dear Family,

We've had a couple close fly-bys at our butterfly garden, but no residency yet. The setup looks so inviting! The Sister says maybe the butterflies come only when we're not looking. Sunday, at church, Linda pressed a cute sticker book (filled with grasshoppers, butterflies, caterpillars, and such) into the Sister's hand. A note attached to the front read: *(Sister's name) Until your butterflies come, use this card garden to dream and believe. Linda.* I hope you're not butterfly haters because the Lady decided to leave Butterfly Weed on our front porch for you. Maybe if we band together we can draw more butterflies to Mansfield. The Dad said not to worry, though, he'll get our garden situated when he gets here.

The Sister had several things she needed to get done before chemo on Tuesday so we drove her around on Monday. The oddest thing happened. She needed to go to her bank and take care of some business so we parked as close as we could to the door. The Lady and I waited in the car listening to KLTY and singing. Because our backs were to the bank's door, the Lady kept looking over her left shoulder to see if the Sister was coming. She didn't want her to have to walk very far since the Sister's so tired all the time now. Anyway, it took a long time before the Sister finally exited the building. When she got in the car, she said they were asking for another I.D. and she didn't have one. The tellers were talking among themselves and then looking at her. It made her uncomfortable. Since it was taking so long, she quietly asked them if there was a problem, but they finally relinquished the cash to her. As we pulled out of the parking lot, the Lady looked over at the Sister. Then it hit her. She knew what the problem was. It was because the Sister no longer looked like the photo on her driver's license. It was a combination of her wig and the dark sunglasses she wore inside and didn't remove. It's a wonder the police weren't called and she was led away handcuffed. We laughed so hard at that scenario we couldn't stop!

Tuesday morning, we entered the cancer center for the long treatment day to begin. After the Sister had lab work done, we sat in the chairs against the back wall nearest the chemo door and watched TV until her name was called. In the vacated chair, the Lady set up our area for the five-hour wait. She carried a navy blue JPS satchel that holds everything we may need—the Sister's medical records folder (which eventually gets so heavy the Lady cleans it out, adding papers to the larger file she keeps in her closet), puzzle and crossword books, a date planner, a bottled water, and for me—a notepad with pens in case I feel like writing home. The next part tells you just how comfortable she is in this environment a year later. Slipping off her tennis shoes, she unzips the side pocket of the satchel and produces a set of footies and places them on her feet. Curling her legs up in the chair, she slips on her reading glasses, checks her cell phone, then pulls out a book. Officially, we're now settled in for the long haul.

The waiting room was barely crowded. We think Tuesdays are going to be much better for long treatments than Mondays. The Sister, hardly gone any time, poked her head out the door and said for us not to go anywhere. She would be out in a minute. They're sending her home. The Lady hurriedly asks why and she says her white blood count is too low for treatment this week.

Two women sit in front of us. The door hadn't closed shut all the way before the one wearing the du-rag whips her head around and anxiously asks if treatment can be stopped for low blood counts. *Apparently* it can. There's huge concern written across her face so we ask how long she's been in treatment and get a reply of a couple times. The woman sitting next to her turns and says, "I'm her sister. I moved here to take care of her." My eyes open wide at the news. She could have stopped right there, I knew their story. I've lived their lives a year ahead of them. The Lady tells them she also moved here to take care of her sister who's been in treatment for over a year now.

"What kind of cancer do you have?" the Lady asks.

The woman speaks rapidly which lends a certain hint of desperation to her voice. She has breast cancer and didn't even know it. (Oh no, another *no fair, no fair!*) "Now the cancer's all over inside me!" the woman said. (We recognize that, as well.) I see her pause to look intently at the Lady to see what she, a seemingly seasoned-cancer-stranger-lady, has to say about this. I held my breath because her eyes clearly asked, *I'm going to be okay, aren't I?* The Lady begins talking to them, telling them their strength comes from God. They pray for His hand to be on the doctors as they oversee her (the Sister's) care, but ultimately? The true healer is Christ.

Driving home, as I listened to the sisters talk on the phone to Donna and the Parents, it struck me how it had never, ever occurred to me the Sister would have the decision of whether or not she wanted treatment taken from her. Treatment dates will never be concrete again, but taken one week at a time, with blood work dictating the next step.

That night I heard the Lady crying in bed. When I asked what was wrong, she said her chest felt so heavy. What is the medical term for when your chest turns so hard and heavy you can barely breathe? Is that the way it feels when people die of a broken heart? She said she'd never have the guts but, right that minute, she felt like picking me up and running through the streets in her nightgown, not stopping until she pounded on your door in desperation. You'd open the door and there we'd stand. Even though you've never met her, you'd recognize the Lady immediately by her eyes. You'd see for yourself what *I'm going be okay, aren't I?* looks like.

Unaware to the Sister, three afternoons in a row the Lady grabbed her car keys and we left the house for a few minutes. Pulling into a gravel circular drive, parking, then wondering if we should go through with this, it was on the second trip to this home that confirmed we *should* do this and this was the right place. Opening the car door and placing one foot on the ground, the Lady reached down to pluck a shiny dime from among the small rocks. It's a wonder she saw it at all except she was supposed to. After our third unsuccessful attempt to talk with whomever lives there, the Lady placed a handwritten note on the garage door asking someone to please call. That call came a few hours later and the woman on the other end introduced herself as Mara. The Lady explains the purpose of the note she'd left and the two women agree that Saturday, at 9 a.m., would be a good time to meet. Mara says she'll have the gate open, a fan running, a chair, and cold water for us. We can take as much time as we'd like and she's really looking forward to meeting us. Ending the call, we tell the Sister a surprise outing is lined up for her on Saturday.

Saturday morning, we drove through the gate and further down to the barn. The Sister got out of the car and smiled over at us as we walked toward the horse stalls with a large bag of carrots. Happiness is written across her face. In the distance we see Mara making her way toward us. The beauty of her as she draws closer is nothing short of striking. We spend time together sharing stories about our lives while petting and feeding the horses. Making our way back to the car and waving good-bye to Mara, we knew we'd been blessed by the very moment itself. God didn't direct us to just *any* house. He directed us to the *right* house—the house with a woman whose heart's of gold.

Sister's Bucket List Entry: Pet (but unable to ride) a horse—√!

Yours,

Frog

♦ ♦ ♦ ♦ ♦ ♦ ♦ ♦

JUNE 24, 2011

Dear Family,

You'd think having that extra week between treatments would've given the Sister a big boost. That wasn't the case at all! By the time we entered the cancer center on Tuesday for her long treatment, the chemo nurse led us over to Dr. Choufani's office instead. When Lou saw the Sister she said, "Have you looked in the mirror lately? You need to go straight to the emergency room!"

Looking back on the week, it seemed nothing was going right. The Sister couldn't eat because of that bloating between her ribs. She took a liking to freezer pops so we'd cut four or five open at a time, placing them in a tall glass so her fingers didn't freeze. She likes the red and purple ones best. The Lady bought gummy vitamins, orange and tangerine juices, and greens (such as spinach) to try to increase her blood count. We made a trip to Saltgrass Steak House to bribe her with a rib-eye steak (for protein) and loaded baked potato, then we swung by The Cheesecake Factory for no other reason than it was time. The Sister must weigh less than 100 pounds now and has taken on a skeletal look. Her cheek bones are more pronounced and a darkening of the skin appears under her eyes. The rest of her hair is coming out in chunks now and doesn't even bother with the courtesy of quietly leaving her head a little here a little there as it's done in the past. She admits she's afraid to touch it any more than necessary. The Lady knew this loss of hair must be *so* before the Sister even told us because neatly packaged hairballs have started appearing in the dryer again. Her eyebrows have decided to follow suit, deserting her. Every morning as she dresses, we hear her coughing and coughing as she struggles to get her breath. The shortness of breath continues throughout the day and is most apparent when she talks. If she has anything particularly lengthy to say, you can hear her run out of breath before sentences are finished.

Her energy has fled. Several times, the Lady told her we must leave early in the morning and walk in the park even if it's just 20 steps before turning around. She's concerned if the Sister stops moving it'll be the end for her. The Sister says she can't do it; she can barely make it through the house. In the morning, she'll brush her teeth then sit on the floor exhausted. When Monday comes, the Sister just sleeps the day through. The Lady circles around her for any sign of wakefulness so food can be pushed her way.

On Tuesday, using the closed toilet seat as a chair, she sits quietly while lifting her arms and legs as the Lady helps her into clothes. Brushing through her wig before setting it in place, then giving the Sister a once-over with the lint roller, we head out the door. It's the best we can do. As we drive down the road toward the cancer center, more than one of us figure it has to be physically impossible for the Sister to have treatment this time and, again, it was.

Fevers come and go daily. The thermometer finds a permanent spot on the small table beside the Sister. We're not used to this. With the old drug, fevers developed a day or two after treatment then vanished until the following treatment. Clothes will be shed and the wig will be removed and placed across the back of the couch. The air-conditioner doesn't help matters and goes on the fritz when a coil freezes up. Shutting down the unit until the ice thaws off the coil, then turning it back on, is a temporary fix. The Lady's oldest son's close friend, Jared, makes an out-of-the-way trip to rescue us and (thanks to the Dad) lines up installation of a new unit.

Where's the blessing in all this? The Brother's second PET scan comes back clear of cancer. The Parents make the long journey here to spend time with us. The oldest nephew cleaned up the Brother's dusty, unused walker so the Lady could take the Sister to her favorite park. She was able to make a complete lap around it with the walker.

We received the following text: *Just found a dime! Wanted to let you know I have thought about you guys every day since we first spoke and will continue to do so! Happy Wednesday! I am in Grapevine at Bostons Pizza! I never find dimes! Crazy! Mara*

Yours,

Frog

◆　◆　◆　◆　◆　◆　◆　◆

JULY 2, 2011

Dear Family,

On Tuesday, the Sister had a doctor's appointment before heading over for another try at chemo. I believe it's become apparent to all who know the Sister, her health is deteriorating. Days are difficult to get through, and nights are finished off with a good bout of crying between the Lady and I. Instead of sleeping, the Lady lies with her eyes closed and comes up with various strategies to try to keep the Sister active. She'll hit her pillow with her fist when she thinks of things she should've promoted stronger or incorporated sooner, then makes a mental list with promises she'll try harder tomorrow. The Sister can't get rid of the fevers that come and go every day. When we arrived in chemo on Tuesday, they ran her vitals. Her heart rate was high and she had a fever so, once again for three weeks in a row, there will be no treatment. It was decided to have a urinalysis and blood taken (from her port site and arm) for testing to see if anything is showing up.

We try every morning to get the Sister up and over to the park to walk so she can gain strength, but Thursday she didn't want to even try so we stayed home. Yesterday (Friday), she only walked a little then collapsed onto a park bench because she was so dizzy and short of breath. The Lady second guesses her decision and worries maybe she's pulling what little strength the Sister has right out of her. We drove back home, letting her know we'll just keep on trying every day. How ever many steps she can take is fine because there are no rules; we don't have to walk the *whole* track. Throughout the day, she flitters in and out of sleep. Days ago, the Sister told us she was too weak to manage using Donna's special big, plush towel anymore. It's too heavy and throws her off balance when she wraps it around her head. She asked us to find the thinnest towel in the house for her to use now.

Ever since last week, when we were sent to the emergency room, the Sister's had really bad pain in her liver area. The doctor pressed around on her stomach, but when he got to her liver and pressed, she yelled out in pain. For two days after that, she had difficulty getting up and down. She walked very slowly stooped over. She says there's a golf ball-size knot in her liver area and doesn't know if it was there before the doctor pressed on her or not because she never felt around that area. The Sister asked the Lady, "Do you have one too?" The Lady laid on the floor and started working the fingers from both her hands in opposite directions around her rib cage, concentrating hard to see if she felt any difference in the right side versus the left. Pressing, pressing, pressing, on and on, until the Sister started laughing. The Lady was hoping she had a knot on her right side so she could announce there's absolutely nothing to be concerned about. She *too* has a knot so, whew, it's all normal!

Since Monday is the 4th of July and the cancer center will be closed, the Lady and I went there Friday morning to find out what time the Sister was supposed to see the doctor on Tuesday. We never got an appointment slip in the mail. The Sister said she doesn't want to know what the next CT scan results are unless it's good news. Also, she doesn't want anyone telling her any timeframe about how long she has to live. So while we were there, we were going to tell Dr. Choufani's staff to mark her records so no one messes up and accidentally lets something slip that she doesn't want to hear. However, it turned out to be an altogether different day than either of us could have foreseen.

We were led to a back office and gently told the Sister's case had been discussed and the chemo is causing more harm now to her body than good. It's killing her. The symptoms are her body's way of saying it can't take any more. It's done now. There aren't going to be any scans or treatments. With those words, the Lady and I draw closer to each other.

"I have to say, more than one person here has mentioned their surprise she's made it this far."

The Lady replies, "Well, (swallowing hard) we're a tough family."

"We want to give her some good days now," Lou, the nurse, said.

They are notifying hospice; it'll be good for the Sister. They'll try and build her body back up, get the chemo out of her system, and make her comfortable. They even had a patient who jumped right back up,

---

after hospice came in, and was able to continue with treatment again. He had stage four liver cancer, and just recently passed away.

The Lady tells Lou, "We can't tell her it's *hospice*. We just can't! We can say it's home health care coming to visit."

"It's not home health care, and all the forms the Sister will have to sign will say hospice, but you could say it's palliative care." Neither one of us even knows what palliative care means, but it does sound better than the "H" word. Lou seems in no hurry to leave the room and stays to comfort us.

Standing up to leave, the Lady hugs Lou. "Tell Dr. Choufani we love him, and I hope you know we love you too."

Lou takes us back to the waiting room and asks us to have a seat while she talks with Dr. Choufani and completes the doctor's orders. The Lady looks lost and I've never seen her so devastated. In front of everyone, she kept grabbing a new tissue after soaking one, holding it over her face, then quietly sobbing and sobbing and sobbing. People kept looking our way with apprehension. Some offered her a comforting look, while others looked frightened, perhaps the difference being whether they were patient or caregiver. Lou returned and, with concern on her face, asked the Lady if she was capable of driving home. Pressing her cell phone number into the Lady's hand, Lou says, "Call if you need me."

When we got back to the house, the Lady sat down next to the Sister and had to refrain from placing the Sister's hand in her own, a sure sign all was not good. She told her they were stopping treatment until her body gets back into shape. A nurse will be coming out to give her palliative care.

"What's that?" the Sister asks.

"It's where they see how they can help you, like maybe give you steroids to get some strength back in you."

"Oh, good! As long as it's not hospice!"

I have a headache. I'm going to stop for today.

Yours,

Frog

◆　◆　◆　◆　◆　◆　◆　◆

　　　　　　　　　　　　　　The Frog Letters

JULY 8, 2011

Dear Family,

Things moved very quickly after hospice was notified. If you've never had any interaction with hospice, which the siblings hadn't, I can tell you they're very efficient. You don't have to do a thing. Within hours of the doctor's orders being completed, the Lady received a phone call from hospice and chose Covenant Care as the provider. Shortly after, Covenant Care called to set up an appointment for a representative to visit the house the following day.

Saturday morning, the Sister woke up and said the world looked yellow. When she opened her eyes, everything had a yellow hue to it. Bending over to rinse her mouth out after brushing her teeth, her head felt too heavy to hold up and she almost lost her balance.

"I don't like what's wrong with me. I feel weird. You're not hiding something from me, are you? Nah! (chuckling) Just kidding!"

We went for a walk in the park and the Sister said not to bring the walker this time. She thinks it's too heavy to maneuver, causing the walk to be more difficult. We make it around the small circle at the park, stopping at every bench along the way to rest, then we came home and the Sister got sick to her stomach.

Covenant Care arrived and explained to us the services they can provide the family. They left a binder for the nurse to use to record information when she makes her weekly visits. Later, the Lady thumbed through it and removed pamphlets and printouts that describe what to look for in a patient's final weeks before death. Not wanting to read this information, yet unable to stop herself, she scanned over it with a sick stomach before hiding the papers in her closet. That afternoon, a medical equipment company delivered an oxygen machine to the house, asking if they were sure they didn't also want portable tanks. "Portable tanks? That won't be necessary," the sisters told him indignantly. (What does he thinks she is? Really *sick* or something?) The machine is just here as a backup. If the nurse ever feels it's needed, it will already be here. It wasn't long before

DianaRae   215

another vehicle pulled up to the house delivering a "comfort kit" from a pharmacy. The kit contains liquid morphine, liquid Ativan, suppositories for fevers and nausea, drops to control saliva flow, and various other meds that may be needed.

For the next three days, the Sister refused most food and lay on the couch, falling in and out of sleep. Tuesday, announcing she wouldn't be putting on any makeup that day, she just felt like lying around. The Lady got choked up, telling the Sister she's very afraid because she's not eating and she needs food to build her body up. The hidden paperwork the Lady read says in black and white not to force patients to eat if they don't want to. The Lady feels this rule surely must apply to *others*. Perhaps at some point her view could change, but not right now. Wednesday, the Sister decides not to walk in the park, but actually feels better and starts eating again. There's a sense of relief until Thursday when she says sharp stabbing pains are shooting through her right shoulder.

The large knot by the Sister's liver is causing pain and she agrees to take half of a morphine pill before bed each night. Having moved a twin mattress next to the couch for her, they make the space nice and comfy with a feathery mattress topper the younger nephew brought home. Telling her to lay down, the Lady fingers the knot to get an idea of what she's been talking about. It's large, about three inches long and two inches wide. From that night on, the Lady chooses to sleep on the couch near the Sister. They fall asleep to the flickering glow of the muted TV, picking fights between each other.

"You'd be a good home health nurse."

"I don't know about *that*…," the Lady says.

"You're so sweet. I think you'd make a *good* one."

"Not as sweet as you. *You're* the sweetest."

"No, you do *everything*. You're sweeter."

"I love you."

"I love you *more*."

"No, I love *you* more."

"YOU, more than YOU!"

"No, YOU, YOU, YOU, more."

Yours,

Frog

♦ ♦ ♦ ♦ ♦ ♦ ♦ ♦

JULY 18, 2011

Dear Family,

"I realize the mistake I made now," the Sister says while lying on the couch last week. The Sister talks in a slow, tired voice directed toward the Lady. "I shouldn't have disguised my fevers before treatments by taking that ibuprofen. I was just so worried they'd put me in the hospital if they saw I was running a fever and I didn't want to go. I didn't know I shouldn't have treatments with a fever. (She pauses. A look of serious thinking masks her face.) And now I've messed my body up and can't go back and redo it. I should've just gone to the hospital! It would've been good for me! I see that now."

Well, how were any of us to know? The Lady and I think about her words often in the week to come as we watch her slowly whither away. Was that *really* what did it? Did having a fever while doing chemo treatments reduce her to a state of… what? Listlessness? No, that's too weak a word. Vegetative state? Too strong. She hasn't had treatments in over a month and we expected the drug to get out of her system by now, followed by a miraculous transformation where bounds of energy would flow through her.

"If I ever get my strength back, I'm not going back to treatment," the Sister adds.

Weak, the Lady tries to persuade the Sister to let the medical supply company bring her a chair to sit on while she takes her showers. The Sister says she'll start taking baths instead. Anxious she might slip, we rush out and buy slip-resistant strips to line the bottom of the bath tub for her. My days aren't spent writing home so much any more as I watch a slowness descend upon this household that even takes a grip on me. These are slow-motion days—days spent sitting on the floor, watching TV, and waiting for the Sister to open her eyes. Refusing food or drink so many times throughout the days, one afternoon the Lady gently shakes the Sister to wake her, "You've got to eat something. I'm worried, honey. (Tears come to her eyes

DianaRae   217

and her voice catches.) Your body can't survive without food, you know?"

"I can't eat. I can't eat anything right now."

"Just take a sip of Gatorade. Here (pressing a small bottle into her hand), just a sip, okay?"

God help us. She sleeps, and sleeps, and sleeps. As we listen to her breathing and study the features of her face, our hearts are gripped with fear. She looks dead. Why are her eyes partially open when she sleeps and her mouth open? Did her chest rise? Dear God, is she even *breathing*? We become paranoid about everything. Any action or any lack of action, sends us snooping around her to investigate the cause. Recalling she could get pneumonia lying down all day, the Lady grabs three pillows and props the Sister up when sleeping. The large knot on her side becomes so painful it interrupts her rest, making her cry out while attempting to find a comfortable position that doesn't exist. One night, the pain is so severe she agrees to three halves of morphine—one half pill every three hours. She doesn't like whole pills. A whole pill of morphine scares her; a half a pill doesn't seem nearly as frightening.

When the hospice nurse comes for the second visit, she's dumbfounded the Sister isn't willing to take her morphine. The nurse says she should be taking the long-lasting kind every 12 hours and the instant-relief kind any time in-between. If it gets horrendous and she needs something fast, the liquid morphine should be taken. The nurses are kind to the Sister. "We want to make you comfortable. What can we do for you? Would you like a social worker to come talk with you or a Chaplain?" Looking at the twin mattress lying next to the couch, "We can get you a really nice, deluxe electric bed in here! Would you like that?"

The Sister doesn't want drugs. She doesn't want social workers. She doesn't want a chair in her shower, and she doesn't want an electric bed. She wants to LIVE. That's all. She wants to live. She turns less talkative toward us and when her eyes *are* open, instead of watching TV, she stares off into space seemingly deep in thought, or she stares at the large, new print the Lady placed over the fireplace mantle.

He will cover you
with His feathers, and
under His wings

you will find refuge.
Psalm 91:4 (NIV)

On Friday, we wake up to find the Sister dressed and sitting up watching TV in the dark. Donna's flying in and the Lady will pick her up at the airport. We have a fairly decent day. The Sister eats what she can and drinks more than usual, lulling Donna into a false sense of normalcy until Saturday turns out to be a repeat of all the rotten days she's really been having—refusing food, refusing drink. "See what I'm talking about?" the Lady whispers to Donna that night as she expresses concern. Donna sleeps next to the Sister to watch over her. The Lady and I retire to her borrowed room that feels like her own now. An hour later, she throws the covers off and rushes out of the room, kneels next to Donna and whispers in the morning she's calling an ambulance. She's going to tell them the Sister's in critical condition. At this news, the Sister opens her eyes and asks in a small voice, "Am I in critical condition?"

"No," the Lady says, even though no one can dispute she certainly looks critical. Her gut says we've *got* to get her into the hospital, into a *real* bed, not just the ER. She needs to get some new blood in her.

"No, I don't want you to call an ambulance. Doesn't that cost a lot of money?" the Sister asks.

After weighing the ambulance idea back and forth, the three sisters make a pact to rise early in the morning and drive to the emergency room.

Yours,

Frog

♦ ♦ ♦ ♦ ♦ ♦ ♦ ♦

JULY 21, 2011

Dear Family,

At 6:30 in the morning, the Lady pulls into a temporary parking spot outside the doors leading into JPS Hospital's emergency entrance. Speaking to the woman behind the check-in desk, we're asked to go to another desk where the Sister's vitals are taken before taking a seat in the waiting area. Moments later, a nurse comes to ask questions and we're ushered straight through to a private bed in the ER. The Lady, afraid records may have been changed in their system to reflect the Sister's a hospice patient now, quickly lets a nurse know the Sister is unaware of this so it doesn't leak out.

Two caring nurses are assigned to the Sister, and it's not long before the doctor comes in to have a look at her. This doctor is very compassionate and recognizes the seriousness of the Sister's condition. Patting her gently on the back with empathy, he lets her know he's going to see what he can do for her. An IV is started and saline solution is drained into her at a rapid rate while blood samples are taken. The doctor returns, saying he's read her history from the cancer center and the last entry shows they were going to do scans on the Sister. He thinks they should go ahead and do scans, and asks the Sister how she feels about that. The Lady reminds the Sister of the times she's mentioned wishing the scans had been done before treatment ended and now she'll know… BUT, at the same *time*, now she'll really *know*. The Sister agrees to the scans.

In true JPS fashion, we're in extreme luck this morning. It's apparent the team of nurses and doctors overseeing her care recognize the Sister's an angel. The doctor returns to let us know blood tests show her white count is at 18k. (That means it went from 1.7, the last reading we were aware of, to this.) There are also white cells in her urine. At first, the Lady thought, *Great! We needed white cells for such a long time and now we've got them!* What the Lady didn't realize, even in the poor deteriorated state the Sister was in (and this just goes to show how amazing the body truly is), her body recognized it was under attack and started producing a massive army of white cells to fight against the enemy. However heroic this sounds, white blood cells showing up in the urine is a warning sign.

Within the hour, the Sister's looking like a whole new person! It's incredible what a large pouch of saline solution can do to turn around a dehydrated body. A nurse opens the door and, speaking to the Lady, tells her the doctor would like to have a word with her. Rising, she follows behind the nurse to a new doctor assigned to the Sister. They want to clarify the Sister does not know she's a hospice patient. They also want to know why she's bringing a hospice patient into the hospital. Well now, there are hospice patients and then there are *hospice* patients. The way the Lady sees it, technically the Sister's a "pretend" hospice patient right now simply because:

A. She's only been under hospice for two weeks and has seen a nurse once a week—or two times total. According to the Lady, "true, bona fide hospice patients" have to see a nurse daily or at least several times a week.

B. There's hardly any medical equipment in the house yet. Again, according to the Lady, "true, bona fide hospice patients" are hanging out in deluxe powered beds all day.

C. And... because she said so.

This is when the truth to the matter dawned on the Lady. The purpose of hospice, probably in the Sister's case, was to help her die comfortably. By bringing her to the hospital, she was asking them to help her live. So, when they asked why she'd brought a hospice patient in, she told them the first thing that came to her mind, the truth, "Because she wants to *live*."

Later, while passing by the nurses' station, the Lady asked if the scans were back yet. The nurse said they were, then quickly bowed her head. Taking this as a bad sign, we chose to continue on to the Sister's room. Donna left for a long time and when she returned, the Lady left for the restroom and was pulled aside as she passed the nurse's station again. When the scans came back, the nurse compared them to the March scans and was alarmed. (Her eyes filled up with tears). She asked the doctor to come look. The Sister's liver was huge; the knot she'd complained about was actually her liver. A new doctor joined us to continue explaining, her tumors had progressed rapidly since March and they showed the cancer had now spread to her lung and spleen. (What's the spleen? The Lady's heard of it before, but where's it located? *What's your purpose, Spleen?*)

"Don't tell my sister. Mark the records not to tell her about it spreading," the Lady instructed.

Returning to the room, the doctor and nurses came back in to let the Sister know she has a urinary tract infection and they're going to start antibiotics now. They also tell her the scans show her liver is enlarged and the tumors are growing. They're going to keep her here for a couple days. We can think of little else the rest of the day—the part of the diagnosis the Sister wasn't told about. The Lady feels she can no longer hide any of this from her—hide away the fact she's really a hospice patient and her cancer is spreading. Calling Lu Ella late in the day for prayer, Lu Ella agrees that the right thing would be to tell the Sister. If it were herself, she'd want to know.

The Lady remembers the words spoken months ago to the Sister, "We're going to fight this together, (Sister's name), you and me (clear throat) . . . to the end." She fumbles through her wallet and opens the folded piece of paper that was given to her weeks ago. Explaining over the phone to Lou, that the hospital's been notified not to tell the Sister about the cancer spreading, the only one authorized is Dr. Choufani. The Lady asks Lou, "Please ask him to come to us; we can think of no one kinder who could tell her."

They settle the Sister into a beautiful new suite on the fourth floor above the emergency room, a step down from ICU. Her new set of doctors and nurses are a compassionate group. As the Sister falls into a deep sleep for the night, Donna and the Lady make their way back to a house that, devoid of the Sister, isn't the same.

Yours,

Frog

♦ ♦ ♦ ♦ ♦ ♦ ♦ ♦

AUGUST 1, 2011

Dear Family,

Late the following day, as the sisters sat together in the hospital room, the door opened and Dr. Choufani entered, taking a seat in an empty chair near the bed. With quiet concern in his voice, he asked the Sister how she's feeling. Reaching up and gently rubbing the large knot on her right side, the Sister explains the pain she's having, the fevers that won't go away, and the infection they diagnosed her with. He allows her to talk uninterrupted, listening intently to what she has to say. He's in no hurry. Of course, none of us who *know* are. In fact, some of us don't want her to *ever* quit talking but, eventually, Dr. Choufani takes over the conversation telling her he believes the fevers are because of the cancer. He then moves on, occasionally clearing his throat in a manner the sisters have come to find endearing, telling her the cancer has spread now.

Half afraid to look, the Lady glances over at the Sister. Silent tears are trailing down her cheeks as she gazes straight at Dr. Choufani, absorbing his words. I can't help but think what a remarkable person she is not to lose control, or weep loudly, or demand they sedate her until she can come to terms with the news. That's all she has to say about the matter . . . silent tears.

He lets the Sister know treatment is stopping and he's placing her under hospice care. "Do you like those people? Have they been good to you?" he asks. She nods yes, they have, and doesn't ask if "those people" were "hospice" before she even came into the hospital. Like everything else in her life, she handles it with quiet acceptance. Dr. Choufani leaves and the sisters huddle together to comfort each other with prayer. Donna decides to stay the night at the hospital with the Sister.

The following afternoon, we took Donna to the airport then drove back to the hospital for the Sister. As they were wheeling her down to the patient loading area, the Lady thought of that morning in the

ER when they questioned why she'd brought in a hospice patient. At that time, there was a male nurse, unassigned to the Sister, standing at the nurses' station writing in a chart. She remembers his casually spoken words, "You can't keep bringing a hospice patient in every time they're dehydrated." She wanted to get defensive, ask him to step forward, announce himself, and proclaim his intentions. As hard as it was to accept, she knew he was right. Someone had to tell her. Someone had to say it. So, as we pulled out of the parking garage and up to the curb to claim the Sister, the Lady knew from here on out her duties would be split. She would have to help her to live, and she would have to help her in death.

The Sister gave up when we brought her home.

Yours,

Frog

♦　♦　♦　♦　♦　♦　♦　♦

AUGUST 3, 2011

Dear Family,

On the second day of her giving up, the Sister pulled herself up out of sleep and carefully picked a route back to her bathroom. As if she were on the lookout for hidden landmines, each step was measured. Each step painfully slow on legs that threatened to no longer support her. We didn't realize what it had taken to make that walk until we went to check on her. The bathroom door was open and, as we peeked around the corner, we saw her sitting on the closed toilet lid. Her upper body was slumped over the counter, with her head resting on her arms.

"Honey? What's wrong?" the Lady asked.

(Slowly lifting her head) "I can't make it back to the couch."

Yelling back toward the living room for the oldest nephew to come help, together they lift the Sister under her arms and settle her back on the couch. The Lady, starting to feel sorry over the whole situation, left the nephew in charge while we headed to the cancer center to see Tricia. She's a Patient Navigator for the American Cancer Society and her office is in Cancer Care Services. This part of the building is a help station for patients where they pre-qualify for treatments, get help with prescriptions, talk with social workers, see if the drug they're going to be on will make them lose their hair, etc. It's been over a year since the time we entered Tricia's office and she asked the Sister if she'd like a wig. "How much do they cost?" the Sister asked. Tricia told her the wigs are free and we left that day with the Sister's first wig, a synthetic one she wore for a long time. Today, for just a moment, we were diverting our attention off the trials at home and giving back by bringing a real hair wig for Tricia to give to someone else. The Lady tells Tricia she's sure she knows the perfect patient to give it to.

It was sad walking through the cancer center without the Sister. It'd been the three of us for such a long time. We wonder if we've made an impact here or if, eventually, we'll be forgotten. Can it ever be the same without these two sisters here? Perhaps there's always *been* a set of sisters walking these halls and, this time, they were the ones to temporarily step in to fill the spot. Maybe the two sisters we met before chemo officially ended *("I'm gonna be okay, aren't I?")* will be the ones who take *their* place.

On the third day of giving up, the Lady called a local Mansfield funeral home to set up an appointment to discuss whatever she needed to know about burying someone. She's never done this before. The Sister's raging fevers have been missing all week and, instead, her temperature has been registering below normal, like 95.6°F or 96.7°F. Researching on the Internet to find out what might cause this to happen, leaves the Lady wishing she hadn't bothered to look it up in the first place. The Sister's stomach is swelling to the point she opts to leave her pants unfastened now. She had to be requalified all over again for hospice care. (Once you obtain care through someone else—the hospital in her case—it releases hospice from their duties and you start the process all over again.) The hospice nurse, Melanie, came to check on the Sister and measured her stomach to begin monitoring the swelling. For having liver failure, they're told, her coloring is good. Her eyes and skin aren't yellow. This prompts the Lady to later research liver failure on the Internet and she notices one of the symptoms is a swollen stomach.

That night, the third night of her giving up, we sat on the floor looking at the Sister while thinking about how fast she was leaving us. *NO! Not today! Not now!* The Lady rose and went to the Sister, shaking her arm until her eyes opened. "You have to eat! I *need* you in my life. (Her voice cracks.) I'll be lost without you." Returning with a warm bowl of chicken rice soup, she begins spooning tiny amounts of broth into the Sister's mouth then adds a few kernels of rice until she estimates five tablespoons have been given to her. It took a lot for the Sister to eat this much and keep it down.

The following morning, the Parents arrive. This is their second trip to Texas in a month to see us. They're worried about the Sister. On this morning, the Sister gets dressed and tries to eat. Her bloated stomach is a problem. She tells us, all those days she slept, she thought she was dying. We told her we thought she was dying too! She said when the Lady shook her arm the night before to wake her, and she saw the stricken look on her face, she realized she wasn't doing anything to help herself and she was going to try again. After hearing that, the Lady thought, *Who do I think I am? If I go to that appointment at the funeral home, it's as good as saying I don't think God can heal her. What a hypocrite I am! He isn't done with her yet!* She hurries and calls to cancel the appointment.

Over the coming week, the Sister begins to gain her strength back. Each day she eats more, and more, and more. The Parents bring her whatever she feels like eating and the Mom makes Cherry Yum Yum, the Sister's favorite birthday dessert, which she hasn't eaten in years. The Dad spends time talking with the Sister and his eyes get watery just looking at her. Out of earshot, he also spends time talking with the two nephews. At the end of a week, the Parents make their journey back home. A renewed hope is blanketed on the household. The Sister has made great strides this week.

Yours,

Frog

◆ ◆ ◆ ◆ ◆ ◆ ◆ ◆

AUGUST 11, 2011

Dear Family,

There are some good things in life—things to rejoice and give thanks about. The Sister's temperature, after weeks of being consistently very low, is registering closer to normal at 98.1°F. The number 98 is a lucky number since her oxygen intake is at 98 percent. Maybe that's why her morning cough hasn't been as bad, and her shortness of breath doesn't make it as difficult for her to talk. Here's the most amazing thing, the feeling has returned to her fingers and feet. We were thinking that was a permanent loss because of the chemo; a lot of times it is.

With nothing left to lose, the Gerson therapy book is dusted off by the older nephew, discussed among everyone, and a conscious attempt is made to incorporate this theory into the Sister's lifestyle. It feels weird using the word *lifestyle*, I mean, what kind of lifestyle is cancer survival? After a trip to the store, we return stocked with fruits and vegetables, and (seven months later) the juicing begins again. The Sister's averaging about four to six cups a day, in 4-ounce servings, of pure fresh juice. This is all she can tolerate. Hating the green vegetable juices, after her second serving she looks ill. That's understandable. Have you ever tried drinking pure lettuce juice without a little Ranch or Italian to spice it up? Adding strong-tasting fruits, such as oranges, help disguise the taste somewhat. Celery is the green juice she hates the least and all the pure fruit juices taste so good it's equivalent to a dessert.

Sunday after church, the Lady starts a pot of Hippocrates Soup. She buys leeks for the first time in her life; holding one up, she thinks, *so THAT'S what a leek looks like. It sounded like it should look more ugly!* The Lady serves the fresh, warm, vegetable garlic soup puree and the Sister likes it. The Lady spends about five hours that day reading through the Gerson book to become familiar with the program. As the Sister spoons the soup away, happy feelings flee when the Lady reads the part about water intake. She screwed the soup up by making the base with tap water and not distilled water.

For breakfast on Monday, the Lady serves the Sister oatmeal with raw honey drizzled on top. The Sister can have as much oatmeal per day as she likes as long as it's plain, cooked oats without any "bells or whistles." (Bells or whistles = instant oatmeal flavored with brown sugar, apple, cinnamon, etc.)

In order for the therapy to be most effective, coffee enemas are suggested. The Sister did this once or twice last year before quitting. Coffee grounds are boiled for 15 minutes in distilled water, cooled to body temperature, then… well, *you* know. On the Sister's first attempt this time around, she was in her bathroom for a long time and we could hear her getting frustrated so we tapped on the door.

"How's it going? Everything okay?"

"The tip's stuck."

"Stuck? (*Where? Oh my gosh, should I call hospice?*) Do you need some help pulling it out?"

"The coffee's not coming out."

"Oh! That's okay! I read about that. They said sometimes the coffee's absorbed and won't come out. Don't worry about that."

"But, it's not coming out of the tip!"

"Open the door. Let me see."

We weren't sure what we'd see when the door opened. The Sister, fully dressed at the sink, was trying to get coffee to flow from the bag, through the line, and out the tip. She hadn't even started "the process" yet. The Lady's never used one of these things and started trying to get the flow started. Once the flow starts, you can clamp it off until it's "time." After a ridiculous amount of time passed, the tube was fed into the bag and pulled back out half a dozen times, but nothing was allowing the coffee to flow through to the tip. Looking at the tip, it looked brand new. Remembering Mechanics 101, the Lady rinsed it under hot water and (trying not to think about it) started ciphering it out with her lips. Hitting the clamp to stop the flow, it worked!

Well, it worked until later that day when it was time for the second dose. The same problem occurred. After fiddling around with the bag and hose, the Sister grabbed the bag and held it upside down, resulting in coffee gushing out into the sink. They bantered back and forth, the Sister saying the bag *has* to be held upside down; she remembered that part. The Lady said for her to have a look—there's a big *hole* at the top. See? That's why coffee is POURING DOWN THE DRAIN when you turn it upside down! Finally having a look, the Sister realized she forgot to get the cap, that seals the top, out of the box. That was the problem all along. The Lady looked at her and said, "Well! I wish you'd remembered the cap *before* I tried sucking on the tip for a SECOND TIME!" We laughed about it while the Lady tried not to dwell on to what extent she's willing to go to help this sister of hers live. She can't think of anyone else she'd ever do that for, probably including herself! Thank God for enema bag caps! I don't even know why I told you that weird story. You won't tell anyone else, right?

Okay, enough of the good news. Let's move on to the not-so-good news and how we camouflage the reality to preserve our sanity.

The Sister has started the shakes in her hands. Twice she's dropped her glass of juice all over herself and the couch. We blame this on the coffee enemas and the caffeine going straight into her bloodstream. Never mind those shakes started before enemas were introduced.

Her stomach continues to bloat and this is due to all that time she didn't eat or drink. This is kind of like what happens to starving children in Ethiopia. Not to worry! This is about to disappear any day, now that she's eating again. Never mind this is a sign of liver failure.

Her ankles are swelling and we can no longer see her ankle bone on one leg, which looks just plain wrong because her legs are so tiny. This swelling is because she doesn't walk much any more.

She's soaking her clothes and bedding with sweat more than ever before. Pillowcases, sheets, and clothes are stripped off and dry replacements found. These are the deadly toxins leaving her body, they agree.

A tiny pill cup is kept on the table by her couch, containing no more than four white halves of morphine (immediate release) at any given time. She can take these throughout the day as needed for pain. Normally, she barely takes two or three halves a day even though she can take four whole ones or more. Two bright blue pills are added to the cup in the morning. These are morphine extended-release pills, which she is supposed to take two a day or one every 12 hours. The Lady always dispenses these and records the time and amount taken so there's no mix-up. It helps the nurse get an idea of when her pain levels are highest and how much morphine she's actually taking on average per day.

On Sunday, the Sister woke up and seemed to be in a state of confusion. The Lady always gives her a Prilosec, a B-12 vitamin, and a morphine ER first thing in the morning. On this day, the Sister announced she'd already taken her morphine and recorded it. The Lady hadn't put the blue pills out yet so she glanced at the notepad where the Sister had written: 7 == 02. Now, 7½ would be the dose for half a white tablet and maybe the 02 is a fancy way of recording she took two halves. When she questioned her, the Sister said she forgot she was supposed to take the blue pill, but she wrote the time she took the white ones. Looking at the pad again, the time she took the pills was 7 == 02. This was the first warning sign that something wasn't right because the Sister's handwriting was way off, as if someone else had written this. The second warning sign came that night while watching TV together in the dark. The Sister started talking softly and making comments that didn't pertain to anything happening on TV... or anything *else* for that matter. I was going to give you examples, but I just don't feel like it. It's hard when I think back.

Monday, she talks quietly, very slowly, and we have to zoom in close to catch what she's saying. Then, pretend we either know what she's talking about or say we weren't paying attention and apologize. It's like she's sitting up awake, but not *here*. So, with the new symptom of confusion added, we tell ourselves it's that darn urinary tract infection she had a couple weeks ago at the hospital. Those infections will mess with your mind.

The Lady and I pull the oldest nephew aside to tell him it seems her confusion started just a few days after they started juicing. He had noticed that too and was going to talk to us about it. What should they do? Are they filtering too many pure nutrients through a non-functioning liver? Is this causing her more harm than good? Also, they keep screwing up and accidentally giving her a banana or using tap water. Besides that, honestly, who has the heart to rip that piece of string cheese out of her hand and deny her? They come to agreement, it's time to let her eat whatever she wants. The Lady, bawling her guts out while discussing this with Donna over the phone, looks for reassurance over this decision. Donna's also in agreement and she'll be flying back here Friday. Hurry up Friday!

The following day, we were the first customers at Saltgrass Steak. They weren't even open yet when we ordered a rib-eye and loaded baked potato to go.

Yours,

Frog

♦ ♦ ♦ ♦ ♦ ♦ ♦ ♦

AUGUST 13, 2011

Dear Family,

We put a call into hospice for Melanie, her nurse, to come early this week to check on the Sister. The nurse thinks the liver tumors might be leaking ammonia into the Sister's system, which causes confusion. Taking her vitals and then looking at her eyes, the nurse wants to know if her eyes look slightly yellow to us. The Lady got up close to look at the Sister's eyes and replied, "No, I can't really see any *yellow...*"

This is a bad day for the Lady. It seems she's looking a little more rough lately. She told me her mind feels foggy and she desperately just wants to sleep. It doesn't seem she accomplishes much around the house and her organized days are scattered with whatever demands dictate. The dishwasher might not be emptied first thing in the morning. Clothes are left in the dryer instead of being folded immediately. Her hands are chaffed from all the times she dissembled the juicer and washed it out in our measly attempt to save the Sister. Hurry, Donna, get here.

The day after the nurse left, the Sister sat up that morning and her voice was different; it sounded weak and shaky. Sitting next to her, she tells us sometimes she doesn't know what we're saying to her and she feels badly when she asks us to repeat ourselves. We tell her to ask as often as she needs to, and if we talk and she doesn't feel like answering, she doesn't have to. We understand. The Sister, with a pitiful, defeated look on her face, starts to cry because she doesn't know what's wrong with her mind; she doesn't understand some of our words now and she can't think of what words are needed communicate. We experience a soul tattoo. What's worse, losing your mind and not even being aware of it or losing it and knowing it's leaving? We can hardly bear this.

The next day, we looked at her first thing in the morning and thought, *Dear God! Her eyes are really yellow. What does yellow mean? I don't like yellow!* Yellow means something in medical terms, but to us? Yellow means she can no longer walk alone or stand on her own. Yellow means she refuses any food or drink—even the tiniest amounts. Yellow means she can no longer swallow her pills and, instead, holds them with cheeks inflated with drink, then refuses to complete the task—the swallow. (Liquid morphine is brought out to use from then on.) Yellow means she doesn't know what day it is any more and asks in a quivery voice, "Is it day or night?"

The following day, when her eyes are turning really *really* yellow, one of the most unbearable things of all occurs when she turns her head away from us if we speak to her. She doesn't want to look directly into our faces and just wants to be left alone. She stares at the TV, but we can't be sure what she's really seeing. While attempting to get up from the couch, and weakly falling back down, the sisters will share their last full conversation between the two of them:

"Where you going? To the bathroom?"

"I got a lot of little bags to throw away. When people come over, I've got a lot of bags to throw away again."

"Those little Walmart sacks?"

"No. Bigger ones."

"Those large trash bags?"

"No. There're branches I need to throw away. You know the ones?"

Having no idea, yet unwilling to cause the Sister stress, the Lady replies, "Yeah. You want me to throw them away for you?"

"No."

"I will! If there's something you want me to throw away just tell me."

"I got a lot of little bags to throw away, when company comes."

"Like Donna? Tomorrow?"

"No."

"Well (rubbing her hand back and forth on the Sister's leg), we'll throw them away together, okay?"

That was Thursday. Thursday, August 11. The 11th day of August. I have to remember that date.

We didn't go to sleep until the early hours of Friday morning. The Sister was on her comfy mattress on the floor near the couch. She lay with her eyes wide open and not blinking. We watched for a blink and she didn't blink. This bothers the Lady so she gently closes her eyes, afraid her Baby Girl's eyes are going to dry out. Placing her hand on the Sister's stomach, she feels it rise and fall in life. Slowly, the Sister's eyes creep back open, but she's no longer with us. Her body is alive, but her mind lives somewhere else now. The older nephew whispers, "I wonder where she's at..." We don't want to miss one minute with her. We're afraid we'll close our eyes, or divert them for just one itty bitty moment, only to open them and discover something's changed forever in that mere instant. The Lady prays for the Holy Spirit to touch the Sister, fill her with comfort and security, hold her hand . . . hold *all* our hands. As we fought against the sleep that was overtaking us, we felt an incredible sense of loss. We were missing the Sister already.

Yours,

Frog

♦ ♦ ♦ ♦ ♦ ♦ ♦ ♦

AUGUST 19, 2011

Dear Family,

Back before things were really *really* yellow, with difficulty, the Sister got up three mornings in a row asking if Donna was coming that day. She'd made it a point to look her best even in her poor, deteriorating state. Giving herself a sponge bath, which made the Lady nervous when she found out, and finishing her look with her wig, she was ready. "Where's Donna?" the Sister would ask. Each day, the Lady would tell her, "Donna's going to be here Friday, not *today* but Friday. Pretty soon Donna will be here."

The household turned desperate in their attempt to help the Sister's faculties return. The Lady called Melanie to see if Dr. Capper would please prescribe Lactulose, a medication that helps eliminate ammonia in patients. The nurse explained this might not be an option, but she'd certainly let the doctor know our request. The Lady can barely speak as she tells Melanie how difficult it is knowing the Sister's aware of what's happening to her mind and to please ask Dr. Capper if there's any way, as a courtesy to the family, he can do that for us. Melanie calls us back, moments later, to let us know Dr. Capper's willing to do this. They understand what we're going through and will give the medication a try to see if it helps. We hang up filled with gladness. It reminds us of the motto imprinted on the outside of the Sister's file: *Covenant Care – Valuing Life at Every Stage.* These people aren't unreasonable at all! They're great and compassionate and fast because a few hours later, the medication was delivered to our door by a pharmacy courier service.

It's finally Friday! As Donna and the Lady embrace at the airport, we can only hope the Sister's aware Donna's here. While driving, the Lady explains what to expect when we get home. She then calls Covenant Care to let them know the Sister's rapidly deteriorating. Filling them in on the details, she tells them how much liquid morphine and Ativan she's now giving the Sister. They ask about the

Sister's breathing and if we'd like a nurse sent over, but the Lady doesn't think that's necessary right now since Donna's a nurse. They call us twice throughout the day, asking how the Sister's doing, also checking on us in case we need reassurance or backup. They tell the Lady they can send a nurse at any time. That's what they're here for, and not to feel uncomfortable calling at any time, even at night. After hanging up, there's no doubt, we aren't going to be alone during this phase.

Getting back to the house, Donna's shocked to see the situation and spends the rest of the day silently crying while taking charge with her nursing instincts. The Lady and I make appearances to check on them and always discover Donna either lying next to the Sister with her hand on her, or cradling her in her arms and whispering sweet words for just the two of them. For the most part, our Baby Girl is somewhere else but, believe me, the God this family's always speaking of is faithful in showing them He's near. I knew this was so when I tried to make out unintelligible words spoken by the Sister, but twice I heard her say, "Donna."

Also, twice on this day, the Lady got her face up close to the Sister's, trying to reach through to her by loudly speaking, "Baby Girl? I love you!" and I saw the Sister silently mouth back, "Love you." Can you see how God continues to say, *I'm there*?

Yours,

Frog

♦ ♦ ♦ ♦ ♦ ♦ ♦ ♦

Dear Family,

Because it seems inevitable now, and wanting to spare the Parents and her nephews the grief of the task, the Lady made an appointment with Blessing Funeral Home in Mansfield. Arrangements are drawn up and discussed. We drive home thinking about caskets and flowers and announcements and obituaries and unfinished bucket lists and a woman's shoe clad toe tapping a spot under a large Texas scrub oak.

Donna takes night duty and makes a pallet next to where the Sister lays. At 3:30 in the morning, she rushes back to the Lady's room, waking her to say the Sister's all over the place! Quickly fastening her house robe, we race behind Donna then look in awe at the sight before us. After days of the Sister being so weak she could no longer hold herself up or even lift her arms, progressing on to a seemingly unconscious state, by the flickering light of the television we now see her sitting up on her knees before the screen. I notice, right away, how straight her back is, how high her head is held, how strong she sits with no help from her sisters. Shocked disbelief races through us; she does this alone.

Spellbound, we stand frozen as we silently observe the Sister. Reaching her hand up, she touches the television screen in a child's wonderment as she tries to capture the flashing lights and movement with her hand. With reluctance for this moment to end, the Lady slowly moves to kneel next to her, speaking soothing words, they lift her up and settle her in bed.

I'm there.

Yours,

Frog

♦   ♦   ♦   ♦   ♦   ♦   ♦   ♦

AUGUST 31, 2011

Dear Family,

The next morning, we woke up at 5:30 a.m. to the sound of rain. With Texas having drought conditions, the Lady tells Donna she doesn't know if the rain is a sign God will bring relief to the Sister today or if it's nothing more than just the south wind blowing up from the Gulf. We laugh. To my amazement and the sister's delight, the Sister is alive.

I notice Donna's nursing skills have transformed the Sister's bed into an easy maneuvering "sheet technique" for lifting the Sister up to change sheets and positions. This was a far cry from the Lady's technique. Granted, the Lady did everything out of love, but a couple times I saw her stand on top the mattress, placing her feet on either side of the Sister, then bending over to take the Sister's waist in her hands to lift and position her. I figured surely she knew what she was doing until I saw the *correct* way—Donna's way.

It's still a difficult morning. From here on out their goal is to keep the Sister comfortable. The morphine and Ativan (for anxiety) are given more frequently. At this point in her life, the final phase of life, she couldn't survive in any comfortable or respectable fashion without either of these drugs.

I look up from writing my letter home when the Sister becomes restless and moans. The Lady goes to her. The Sister's eyes are open, but I don't think she's with us and neither does the Lady. However, in case we're wrong, the Lady gets down on her hands and knees and places her face so close to the Sister's that their noses almost touch. In a whisper, I hear, "I love you, Baby Girl. (Pausing to see if she gets a response, silence and I remain her only audience.) I love you big as the world, tall as the sky, to the moon and back, from the tips of your toes, and everything in-between . . . "

Yours,

Frog

♦ ♦ ♦ ♦ ♦ ♦ ♦ ♦

SEPTEMBER 8, 2011

Dear Family,

    With the exception of a second pot of coffee being started, there's little activity in the house this Sunday morning. There's not going to be any more Sunday mornings watching the sisters get ready for church, with the Lady grabbing a small bottled water and running the lint roller over the Sister's pants, as we head out the door. There's not going to be any front passenger door opening for the Sister to climb in as the Lady slips her Bible in the backseat. Nor will KLTY be playing as the three of us sing on the way to church. There'll be no more greetings from the friendly man at the door, asking the Lady if he can shake the Sister's hand this week. No more waiting to see what revelation Don will direct toward the Sister, nor a small whisper of a woman seeking the heads of two special women in her life. The Lady won't stand and raise her arms in praise then reach down to quickly pat the Sister's leg as she sits with her own arms raised. No small secret sips of water will be given as another watches on with a kind smile. Driving home, we won't ever discuss between the three of us what great thing the pastor had to say, or agree how beautiful his wife looked. The Lady will never again turn toward the passenger seat to ask, "Where do you wanna stop this time? Mimi's? Sonic? Luby's? Oh, what about Subway?"

    On this Sunday, God is aligning the members of this family from one coast to the other. He's strategically placing His children among others who will help them today.

    The Brother is far away, visiting his daughter who's pregnant again. He sits outside drinking coffee, while remembering the huge cloud he saw the night before. It looked just like an angel with huge wings, praying. It's a beautiful, calm morning; it's the type morning the Sister would want to be sitting outside, he thinks.

    Here at the house, Donna keeps watch over the Sister as the Lady gets dressed for the day. They'll switch places with Donna heading to the back of the house. The Lady will sit on the floor and place one of the Sister's hands between both of her own. Listening to the constant clicking sound from the oxygen machine, she spends a moment doing nothing more than staring into the eyes of the Sister. Getting an overwhelming feeling the Sister would ask this, if she were able, in a cheerful voice the Lady promptly answers the unasked question, "It's Sunday! Your favorite day!" Within moments, the Sister's breath becomes noticeably more difficult to draw. Leaning far over, stretching out her arm, the Lady quickly shuts off the television's volume. Every ounce of attention will be directed to the quick shift in breathing. Study. Study. Concentrate. Concentrate. Donna, appearing in the distance, looks at her serious expression then rushes back to the Lady's side.

"Oh . . . it won't be long now," Donna says.

The Lady will rise and go back to gently shake the younger nephew awake. "Sweet cakes? It's time." He slowly rolls over to bury his face in his pillow. "Come," she says. Seeking out the older nephew, who's speaking to the Brother over the phone, she'll hand motion him to follow her.

I watch as four of the people who love the Sister most in this world will fall on their knees and gather on both sides of her. Hands will hold her hands. Others will slowly trace a palm upon her legs.

At 10:39 a.m., a text will come through on the Lady's phone from Lu Ella's husband, Ken: *Good Sunday a.m. to you dear ones. Having a prayer meeting tonight, and you all are first on my list. Love you!*

At church, Linda's husband will turn to her and comment he doesn't see the sisters.

On the east coast, the Mom and Dad, surrounded by people who love them, will leave church and sit down for lunch with their friends Ken and Joann.

Here, the family waits for each breath the Sister can produce. They are slow, long-drawn breaths from deep within her now. We silently wait to see if she can muster up the strength for the next one. Feeling convinced each breath before must have been her final one, we're constantly surprised and relieved when we hear the next one gradually forming.

Looking at the time on his phone, it's nearing eleven in the morning. The Brother will take a sip of coffee, look up, and watch the most beautiful yellow butterfly flutter by. He'll think about how the Sister would love to see this and how much he loves her.

DianaRae

Donna whispers to the Sister, "Don't be afraid that you're shy. He won't let you go alone. Grandma and Grandpa will be waiting for you."

Waiting on edge, extra long seconds tick past this time. All— still poised and hopeful. All—as expectant as they were with every single breath taken for the past 30 minutes. Truthfully, becoming so familiar with the pattern by now, the mere odds seem in favor this will continue on. There will *definitely* be another breath; surely, there will be . . . That next breath never *does* come. There's only silence, just . . . silence, because none of us are willing to be the first to voice, *"She's gone!"* because of that one rule. Yeah, as long as you don't say it out loud, it isn't so.

Expectancy is replaced with confusion and then with a feeling of . . . a feeling of . . . *We've been tricked!*

The scene before me turns indescribable because it doesn't involve sight, but a very real atmospheric change occurring in the air around us. No movement, none whatsoever in this room, but *still* a physical changing within the very air we breathe. We all feel it—every single one of us. No *one* particular aspect of it is any stronger nor occuring any sooner, it arrives and plays out in an asssemblage of instantaneity. An incredible concurring of calmness, peace, contentment, holiness, a lifting up, a spiritual leaving, a releasing, a confirmation, a speaking to hearts that's so tangible and concrete you're absolutely convinced were you to throw your hand into the air you could feel it—all *this* that blankets us, brush against our skin.

One second you're feeling it, and the next, you're feeling it dissipate as it rises upward and is gone—completely gone. Even goneness feels physical, like a sort of parting kiss tucked inside the passing, leaving with it knowledge of what could never be spoken aloud. *She's gone.*

I quickly throw my head up. Worried for the Lady, it's her face I seek now. In the moment my eyes fall upon her, she bolts to her feet as if attempting to rejoin the goneness before it's unattainable. Donna quickly reaches out to still her as a broken half-scream half-cry of anguish invades our silence.

"Angels stand with her!"

Love,

Frog

◆　◆　◆　◆　◆　◆　◆　◆

The Frog Letters

Gone from My Sight

I am standing upon the seashore. A ship at my side spreads her white sails to the morning breeze and starts for the blue ocean. She is an object of beauty and strength. I stand and watch her until at length she hangs like a speck of white cloud just where the sea and sky come to mingle with each other.

Then someone at my side says: "There, she is gone!"

"Gone where?"

Gone from my sight. That is all. She is just as large in mast and hull and spar as she was when she left my side and she is just as able to bear the load of living freight to her destined port.

Her diminished size is in me, not in her. And just at the moment when someone at my side says: "There, she is gone!" There are other eyes watching her coming, and other voices ready to take up the glad shout: "Here she comes!"

And that is dying.

(Henry Van Dyke)

I'd like to express thanks to the hundreds who gladly posed with the Frog during the course of our journey. I treasure every picture and the memory that goes with it and it's unfortunate I was later unable to locate many who posed with the Frog.

It's with regret I was unable to include the hundreds of pictures surrounding the Frog in this book as well as the letters and pictures involving the Frog Twin's visit to Suwanee, Georgia. It could never diminish in my heart how truly special each of you are.

Video link: http://www.youtube.com/watch?v=MtqHVcnm0Kc

Please visit link to view many of the individuals who posed with the Frog.

ACKNOWLEDGMENTS

My most sincerest and heart-felt thanks to:

The Frog's family—for letting me borrow the Frog and providing me a therapeutic outlet of sharing our story with strangers. Much love and thanks for giving me the gift of time, the time needed to heal.

Oceans and oceans of love to Dick and Sandy Snyder, my parents—my biggest cheerleaders.

Dr. Elie Choufani, Dr. Juan Carlos Hernandez, Dr. Yadro Ducic, and John Peter Smith Health Network; Dr. John Mahoney, Dr. Jeffrey Kneisl, and Carolinas Healthcare System—for exemplifying outstanding excellence in your medical fields.

The countless who became part of our journey—the pieces of our story, family, friends of our family, old friends and new—for giving us treasured memories and an abundance of support. Each and every one of you are a light.

North Gwinnett High School, Suwanee, Georgia, students and staff; Gwinnett County, Georgia, Relay For Life; Tarrant County, Texas, Relay For Life—for rallying to give my sister a chance to celebrate another birthday. I still get choked up at the gesture.

High Point Church, Arlington, Texas; Pleasant Valley Baptist Church, Indian Land, South Carolina; the nation-wide churches and prayer groups who lifted our family up—as Lu Ella would say, to God be the glory!

Henry at CVS Pharmacy, S. Cooper Street, Arlington—you were always a bright spot during the hundreds of trips I made for picture purposes.

Nancy Konopasek—for the professional advice, sound suggestions, and editing provided.

Bryan Howard—for doing a superb job in restoration of the frog photos.

Janine Smith/Landailyn—for bringing the cover photo to life with her talent and skills.

Logan Gilpin/Under the Tower Productions—there *are* no words! Your vision for the book trailer video far surpassed what I could've hoped for.

Note to the Reader

When you give, it's so much more than walking canes being tossed aside, PET scan results coming back clear or final treatments. It's about giving two sisters another day together.

In Memory of The Sister
Covenant Hospice & Palliative Care
3221 Collinsworth St., Suite 160
Ft. Worth, Texas 76107

*

In Memory of The Sister
John Peter Smith Cancer Center
Attention: Administration
601 West Terrell
Ft. Worth, Texas 76104

About The Author

DianaRae currently resides in downtown Fort Worth, Texas. She's the mother of three wonderful adult children and "Nonie" to her first grandchild, Adaline. She enjoys walking around Sundance Square and attending local plays as well as dining with members of a supper club or the special women at CCFW .

And yes, she continues to keep her eyes open for shiny dimes, Monarchs, and her prince.

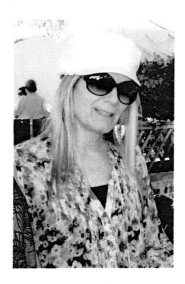

Please send correspondence to DianaRae at:

P. O. Box 7101
Ft. Worth, TX 76111

Or email - diana-rae@hotmail.com

CPSIA information can be obtained at www.ICGtesting.com
Printed in the USA
LVOW12s2204180214

374287LV00002B/89/P

9 781595 945068